Jim

ok.

Bob.

The
ABC's
of the Big

My Life

on Dialysis

BOB NORTHAM

ISBN-13: 978-1477574263
ISBN-10: 1477574263

To Donna.
For her love, support, and,
of course, her editing.

Table of Contents

Preface

Hello. Bob here.

I'm a guy in my late fifties as of this writing, and I lead a pretty normal life.

Except for one thing. I'm on dialysis.

And, I'm a pretty typical dialysis patient.

Oh, again, except for one thing. I tend take a *humorous* point of view of the ridiculous circumstances that dialysis puts me in.

Don't get me wrong, people are only on dialysis because their kidneys don't work, and that's serious business.

My description of what's involved with dialysis treatments and living with kidney failure will show that the potential complications and lifestyle implications are pretty vast. Almost every phase of a dialysis patient's life is impacted by kidney failure and the need for this treatment.

As such, only someone with a sense of humor that's a little off-kilter would find something funny about the whole situation.

So, here I am.

Just to tell you a little more about myself, I'm married with two grown children—a son and a daughter—and one grandson. I just recently retired from my job as vice president of finance for a large corporation.

I initially went on dialysis in my midthirties, got a kidney transplant (the organ was donated by my mom), and went back on dialysis in my early fifties. In total, I've been on dialysis for almost seven years as of this writing.

In that time, I've probably encountered everything that's right and wrong about a life on dialysis, and some of it is pretty crazy.

So, I hope you find this effort helpful, informative, and entertaining. I'm hoping fellow dialysis patients will feel something of a "group therapy" element, and that non-patients will have a feel for what life is like for a person on the "Big D."

I don't mean to explore every angle of every issue—just the ones that we all should be laughing about instead of fretting over.

Sometimes, dealing with these issues is just a matter of perspective...

Introduction

What is this Book about?

This book is about the challenges faced by a person who needs kidney dialysis treatments to live.

Whoa. That sounds way heavier than I wanted it to.

While people on dialysis do face special challenges, I want to bring across that, in many other ways, we're just like other individuals. We have lifestyle issues, work issues, love issues, and time issues. In other words, as my daughter would say, "We have issues."

Some of these issues, but not all, are specific to our needs for these treatments.

For those of you among the uninitiated, I will describe the dialysis process: what it is, why we need it, etc.

I'm hoping that, in some small way, this book will be interesting, informative, helpful, and entertaining. I'm hoping that many of you who are on dialysis will see some commonalities here. And if you can take something away from reading about the way I deal with these life issues, all the better.

And, I would certainly like to hear from readers about other ways to cope with the circumstances associated with life on dialysis.

Should I Expect to Get Medical Advice?

No, do not expect to get medical advice. All I can do is discuss what has worked for me and hope you can gain some perspective from that.

Hey, I'm on dialysis here. Looking to me for medical advice would be like hiring the treasurer of Greece as your personal financial advisor.

Although, aside from kidney failure, I'm generally pretty healthy; the fact that my kidneys don't work puts my overall health assessment in the train-wreck category.

So, please don't make any changes to your health practices or lifestyle based on what I do. Please check with your doctor first.

Is this Book all about Dialysis?

No, droning on about dialysis issues for the length of an entire book would make me want to jump off the nearest cliff. I can't imagine anyone wanting to read an entire liturgy of dialysis this and dialysis that.

I have interspersed some real-life occurrences and general asides to break up the mood.

What's So Funny?

You'll quickly notice that I take a somewhat irreverent view of a pretty serious situation, and this goes against the general consensus that there's nothing funny about being on dialysis.

Horse hockey, I say.

I know, the treatment itself is about as much fun as falling out of a tree.

But, sometimes, if we look hard enough, we can find humor in situations that would make a "normal" person want to run for the hills.

One of my medically non-certified prescriptions for living with dialysis is that we dialysis patients have to laugh every chance we get. This includes even laughing at ourselves, as we often find ourselves in somewhat crazy circumstances.

A dialysis patient's need for treatments can tend to overwhelm the rest of his or her life. I'm a firm believer that if we take a moment to look at the lighter side of dialysis, it will help us on an ongoing basis.

That's my story, and I'm sticking to it.

Lighten Up...Please

Being on dialysis is a serious issue. I know that as well as anyone.

I don't mean to make light of that in any way.

Well, okay, I take that back.

I mean to make light of that in *every* way.

Please don't get offended by my opinions and positions on dialysis-related (or other) issues. Again, the objective is to show how I manage not to take my circumstances so seriously.

If, in some small way, this book can help your mental well-being (MWB) or outlook on life, then it will have been well worth the effort.

Enjoy.

Dialysis Basics

The Initiation

I knew I was in for trouble in my first meeting with a therapist.

When I found out that I was going to need four-hour treatments three times a week, I was a somewhat unresponsive audience. But more on that later.

Put simply, dialysis is a treatment for people whose kidneys no longer function. The kidneys perform the vital function of cleaning impurities out of our blood as well as maintaining a proper balance of fluid and electrolytes in our bodies. A dialysis machine acts as an artificial means of replacing the kidneys' function.

The process is really a medical miracle, although sometimes when you're on these machines for long periods of time, you get the urge to unhook yourself and push the damn thing out into oncoming traffic.

I won't get into a lot of the technical specifications. You may choose some online research to overwhelm yourself with dialysis minutiae at your own risk. But, needless to say, dialysis technology has really improved over the years.

When the concept of replacing kidney function through artificial means first came about, doctors were using every method they could think of, including sausage casings and washing machines. That makes me think of some jokes about beer, brats, and the spin cycle, but we won't go there just yet.

The first attempts at dialysis were taking as long as twenty-four hours. Now, patients can get treatments hooked up to a dialysis machine/artificial kidney in as "little" as three to four hours, three times a week.

Still sounds like a lot of time, right?

Well, it is. When you think about it, the dialysis process is replacing a function that takes place twenty-four hours per day, seven days per week in a person whose kidneys are working normally. And, someone on treatment three times per week is going as long as two days without having any impurities removed from his or her blood.

Given those circumstances, you can understand why a dialysis patient has to live with some restrictions. We can't just live the "normal" lifestyle, eating and drinking whatever we want in between treatments. Besides, as wondrous as the dialysis process is, it is not a perfect replacement for normal kidney function.

The dialysis process does not clean some elements, like potassium and phosphorous, as efficiently as real kidneys. And, since buildup of these elements can be toxic, dialysis patients have to control their intake. I'll describe some of the implications of that later as well.

Additionally, this process doesn't replace some of the critical endocrines normally produced by the kidneys, so these endocrines may need to be added via injection during the treatments.

So anyway, when my kidneys first stopped working, I was a pretty sick puppy, and when I first went to the hospital, I really didn't know what I was up against.

In order to run blood through a machine to be cleaned and balanced, there needs to be an access to the bloodstream. Makes sense, right? Blood has to be removed, treated, and then put back.

Okay, now you're probably all having visions of vampires and zombies.

That's kind of where my mind went during some of my first meetings with the unfortunate hospital therapist the hospital sent in to fill me in on the basics.

Before I had a more permanent "access" to be used for dialysis, I had a temporary catheter surgically placed in my upper chest. The piece was inserted in an artery and had two six-inch tubes sticking out, making me feel like a cross between Frankenstein's monster and Dozer the Gobot.

My therapist calmly explained that, while the catheter was fine as a short-term solution, a more permanent access for treatment would be necessary. Long term, the treatment would be accomplished by sticking two *fifteen-gauge needles* into my arm for every dialysis session.

I sat there calmly nodding, but in my mind I was thinking, *"You're going to do what!?"*

I started picturing myself running down the hall in my hospital gown with some crazy person chasing me with these garden-hose-sized daggers.

As it turns out, that image wasn't too far from reality, aside from the chasing part.

There are several different types of dialysis, but it was determined early on that hemodialysis would be best for me, so that's what the therapist was describing for me.

She went on to explain that the dialysis process involves removing your blood from one of the needle insertion sites to the arterial tube, running it through a semipermeable membrane in the artificial kidney, and then combining it with a solution that removes impurities.

She stopped and asked me what I thought so far.

I said that overall, I'd rather be in Cleveland.

She ignored that and went on.

Once the blood is cleaned, it is then returned to your body through the venal tube and the other needle insertion.

Well, okay, I thought, that doesn't sound so bad, still not knowing, of course, how long the process was going to take or how often I would have to have it done.

Apparently, she was saving these prize revelations for later.

When I asked about the duration of the treatment, she saw me turn a little green when she answered between three and four hours per session.

And I was downright asparagus-like when she said the treatments took place three times per week.

This is one of the most life-changing aspects of living on dialysis. Dialysis patients need these treatments to stay alive, and it's not like putting a mouth guard in at night and forgetting about it. Having to work and live around our scheduled treatments and managing our lifestyles is almost a full-time job in itself.

The time required to get this done right does put a huge dent in our social, work, and life calendars. That was becoming clearer to me the more this conversation went on.

The therapist started getting into some of the more technical aspects of the treatment, but I think she could tell that I was tuning her out more and more and that perhaps I was getting a little overwhelmed with all the implications.

So, she wrapped up the first session but promised to be back later, ignoring the rolling-eyed, "oh boy!" look that I gave her.

I had a feeling that my initiation was only just beginning, and was I ever right about that.

Restrictions

Life on dialysis involves a large number of "restrictions"— things patients can't do that are routine for "normal" people.

The number of dietary restrictions is particularly onerous, as I started finding out in my next couple of sessions with the therapist.

Now, I'm providing the *Cliff Notes* version of these therapy sessions here, but they were really marathon affairs with this poor person loading layer after layer of ways that life was going to change now that I needed the Big D.

I say poor person, because after a while, I was becoming something of an unreceptive audience as the weight of all this change was bearing down on me.

In one of these sessions, she was talking about fluid restrictions.

Fluid restriction is obviously a very important topic. People whose kidneys aren't working properly need to watch their fluid intake because their bodies don't clear fluids as efficiently as others. A person with healthy kidneys will clear excess fluid mostly through urination.

(I'll talk more about peeing later. Can't wait, huh?)

With kidney failure, or kidneys that aren't working properly, fluid can build up in the heart and lungs, resulting in some pretty dire consequences.

The dialysis process clears excess fluid in addition to cleansing the blood.

The therapist was explaining all this and describing how I was going to have to restrict my fluid intake in between treatments. She defined fluids as everything you drink, of course, but also anything that is liquid at room temperature, like ice cream and gravy.

Then, she droned on about how dealing with being thirsty because you can't drink as much as you used to is an ongoing part of life now—yada, yada, yada.

I was getting kind of tired of the whole conversation, and a little overwhelmed by the circumstances in general, so at first, I just gave a little cough.

She thought nothing of it and just continued her onslaught of bad news.

So, I coughed a little more. Then a little more after that.

"Are you okay?" she asked.

"Oh, yeah, just fine," I said.

But, when she started her spiel again, I started choking in earnest and signaled that I needed some water.

Being the good little medical professional that she was, she hurried over to the sink, grabbed a cup of water, and rushed it back over to me.

I acted helpless, so she put the cup up to my lips.

At that point, I stopped the choking act and said in a very calm and professional-sounding voice, "You know, you really shouldn't force water on someone when you're talking about fluid restrictions."

She just looked at me, rolled her eyes, put the water away, and continued the lecture.

Later on, I was able to get a peek at my chart, and I saw the notation "Difficult Patient."

Can't imagine what made her say that.

There are many other dietary restrictions that impact what dialysis patients eat and drink on a daily basis.

Two of the most important restrictions involve foods high in *potassium* and those high in *phosphorous*.

The reason that levels of potassium and phosphorous are important is that the dialysis process does not remove these elements as efficiently as normally functioning kidneys do, which can cause a buildup in the system—not a good thing.

Potassium is a necessary part of our diet, and, in fact, is one of the most common elements found in our bodies.

But like love, children, watching *The Price is Right*, and buying lottery tickets, too much of it is not necessarily a good thing.

In fact, buildup of potassium can cause serious health problems, including death.

I was kind of dosing off when my therapist's lecture hit that last note, but the death part made me sit up straight and start paying more attention.

Because our kidneys aren't clearing potassium normally on a twenty-four-hours-per-day, seven-days-per-week basis, dialysis patients have to restrict the intake of high-potassium foods.

For me, the biggest downside of this restriction was having to reduce or eliminate some of my favorite foods like tomatoes, bananas, potatoes, and oranges.

There is also a lot of potassium in things like avocados, parsley, milk, chocolate, and bran. This is by no means a complete list, and dialysis patients know they have to check the potassium content of anything before ingesting it.

Some processed foods have potassium *added*, which can be really dangerous.

As the therapist was continuing her diatribe, I stopped her and said, "Hey, can we back up a couple of miles and go back to the death part?"

As it turns out, potassium affects muscle contractions, and, since your heart is a muscle, a buildup can actually cause your heart to stop beating.

She said this as calmly as if she was talking about a problem with split ends, but when I gave her the "*Are you serious?*" look, she stopped and said yes, this was legit.

Obviously, potassium intake is not something to screw around with.

After hitting me with the fear of immediate death, the discussion on phosphorous started out a little more calmly.

Phosphorous buildup, while not posing the immediate consequences of potassium buildup, can be just as serious, if not more so, on a long-term basis.

Now, keep in mind that I was still a layman in terms of learning about all these elements when these conversations were taking place. To a layperson, phosphorous sounds like something you might shoot up in a flare gun, but it doesn't mean anything from a dietary perspective.

So, when she brought up phosphorous, I was like, "What kinds of foods have phosphorous in them?"

"Everything," she said.

"Ah. So, I just have to restrict my intake of…everything?"

"Well, sort of."

There *is* phosphorous in just about everything we eat, but as you might expect, some foods are higher in phosphorus than others.

And, though phosphorous may seem like some obscure little, nutty-professor-type thing, it's actually the second most common element found in our bodies after calcium.

And, as I mentioned earlier, the consequences of a phosphorous buildup in your body are not pretty.

My therapist started out with a somewhat technical discussion, explaining that too much phosphorous can cause *hyperphosphatemia.*

She looked like she was expecting me to know what that meant, but I think my eyes glazing over told her otherwise.

Then she said, "Short term, hyperphosphatemia can cause joint pain, bone disease, severe itching, and heart disease."

That perked my attention a little bit more. Of course, as soon as she mentioned itching, I started getting itchy just about everywhere.

"You said short term," I said, scratching under my armpit. "What about longer term?"

She hesitated before answering, as if she was trying to think of a more tactful approach than the ton-of-bricks potassium discussion.

But then she blurted it out, "Well, it can cause your organs to calcify and lead to death."

I just sat there looking at her, thinking, well, here we are, back to death again.

"In fact," she continued, digging in a little bit more, "high phosphorous is one of the leading causes of death among dialysis patients."

Oh boy.

For dialysis patients, controlling phosphorous is difficult because it is in so many different kinds of foods and is commonly used as an additive in many processed foods these days.

Just our luck, it seems as though some phosphorous additives are used to enhance the texture, body, and flavor of a lot of foods, further guaranteeing that what we *can* eat will be taste-free.

Because phosphorous is prevalent in so many foods, most dialysis patients, in addition to limiting/eliminating foods high in phosphorous, have to take a *phosphorous binder*, which is a medication that decreases the absorption of phosphorous into the blood.

The binder that I take is a one-thousand milligram horse pill that I chew along with every meal. The taste is somewhere along the lines of raw baking soda and blackboard chalk.

Some examples of high phosphorous foods that were painful for me to eliminate include cheese, Coca-Cola, hot dogs, beer, and whole grains. Most dairy products are high in phosphorous, and, as mentioned earlier, many processed foods include phosphorous or a phosphate derivative. It is really a good idea to check the ingredient list of *any* processed food that you buy and beware of any word containing "phos" near the beginning of the list.

Most brands of prepared pancake mix, biscuits, waffles, refrigerated bakery products…let's see, anything else in the indescribably-delicious category come to mind?…are all high in phosphorus.

Of course. They just would be.

Just in case there were still some good-tasting foods left that were still eligible for consumption by dialysis patients, there's still one more major restriction category to consider—**sodium**.

Yes, that should just about take care of everything else that I liked to eat before going on dialysis.

The basis for the sodium restriction is twofold.

Excessive sodium intake can raise blood pressure. That statement is true for everyone, not just dialysis patients, but dialysis patients frequently have blood pressure problems to begin with.

And, as my therapist explained to me, sodium has another undesirable side effect for dialysis patients.

It makes you thirsty.

Oh, sorry. I forgot, we're talking about dialysis patients here. I meant to say, it makes you thirst<u>ier</u>.

Since all dialysis patients have fluid restrictions, we're always walking around in a constant state of thirst anyway.

Sodium just makes it worse.

Controlling sodium intake is no small effort. But, I've found over the years that controlling my sodium intake is the key to keeping my fluid gain between treatments under control.

Later in the book, we'll have a whole discussion of fluid intake, thirst, weight gain, and quality of dialysis treatment. They are all related.

So let's say you're an innocent, unsuspecting person just minding your own business when one day you discover that you need to go on dialysis.

(I know it doesn't work that way, but just play along, eh?)

Say your favorite dinner on Saturday night is pizza and beer. You discuss this delicious meal with your new best friend, your dialysis nutritionist. She would point out a few little issues with your meal plan.

Pizza:

- You can't have tomato sauce…too much potassium.

- You can't have cheese…too much phosphorous.

- Toppings? Forget it. Probably too much sodium.

Beer:

- You can't have beer…too much phosphorous. (Not to mention the fluid gain, especially if the first one tasted so good that you decided to have another, or ten.)

- That means your new Saturday night dinner would consist of…pizza dough.

- Oh, but don't buy the premade kind; there's probably too much phosphorous in it.

Now, many of my dialysis compadres have pointed out that you don't necessarily have to completely restrict these dangerous food types, but you should just use portion control.

I've never subscribed to that philosophy. I think that if you dabble here and there you're going to continue to have problems with your potassium, phosphorous, and fluid weight gain. So, I have abstained from the prohibited food groups in their entirety.

Hey, I'm not saying this is easy. I used the pizza example because pizza *was* one of my favorite foods. When one of those pizza ads comes on TV, I'm practically groveling on the floor so close to the TV that I can count the pixels in every piece of pepperoni on the screen.

And beer? Don't even talk to me about beer. The thought of a frosty cold one on a hot summer day? I'd walk around clucking like a chicken for a week if that's what it took to be able to have a couple.

Maintaining your diet is a critical part of not just surviving but thriving on dialysis. I believe in completely abstaining from all foods and drinks that are restricted. Keeping your levels in line is no laughing matter; your life literally depends on it. It's not fun, but neither is kidney failure.

We'll have much more on dietary restrictions and related lifestyle changes further on in the book.

In-Center Hemodialysis

That description probably sounds about as much fun as it is.

Not very, in other words.

There are several different types of dialysis treatments that can keep you alive with kidney failure. For me, the least of all evils is in-center hemodialysis, which, for simplicity's sake, we'll refer to as ICH. (I really didn't mean for this acronym to be spelled as I-C-H, but lo and behold, it turned out that way.)

In order to get this kind of treatment, you have to go to a dialysis center (hence the name.) The center is a small medical building staffed by attendants and a nurse who carry out your treatment.

Another treatment type is home hemodialysis, where your treatment takes place…well, you know.

As I see it, there are two big advantages to going to a center rather than staying at home.

Number one, the attendants and the nurse are trained to respond if something goes wrong during your treatment. Leaving an emergency situation up to me would be a dicey proposition, at best. One time I was changing a fuse at home and almost burned my house down.

Number two, in-center dialysis machines are faster, so you don't need treatments as often.

Typically, an in-center dialysis patient needs three treatments per week. Each treatment can last between three- and four-and-a-half hours. If you choose home hemo, you need six, count 'em, six treatments per week. As in, only one day per week with no treatment. Ugh.

In fairness, there are a lot of patients who choose home hemodialysis, and most of them swear by it.

One of the advantages of home treatment is that your dietary restrictions aren't as prohibitive, since your blood is being cleaned more often.

One guy who was on home treatment was regaling me with how he could now eat all the cheese, Italian food, pizza, and chocolate that he wanted, and all of his blood test readings were still okay. I just smiled, nodded, and said, "Hey, that's great," but down deep, I wanted to reach down his throat and rip his heart out.

Whoops. A little passion coming through there. Sorry.

The choice between in-center and home hemodialysis has trade-offs for sure. My choice has been influenced by the reality of having to depend on a machine to stay alive, and psychologically, it's important for me to separate my dialysis life from my non-dialysis life at home.

The other main type of treatment is peritoneal dialysis (PD), which uses a membrane in your own abdomen to clean your blood. It is done at home.

In order to do PD, you would need to have a catheter inserted into your abdomen—an option that I found particularly unappealing. Long term, these catheters have a high rate of infection, which about sealed my decision early-on.

The Needles

At first, ICH didn't seem too bad to me, relatively speaking, of course. Part of the reason was that, when I first had to go on it, they were using that two-headed monster catheter in my chest to carry out the treatment.

While having the catheter in was hardly ideal, it had the advantage of not involving any needles. The catheter, however, is only a short-term solution. Dialysis doctors don't want to leave catheters in your body too long because the chance of infection is high.

At the same time the catheter was put in, the doctors did surgery on my arm to create what's called an *arteriovenous fistula*, or AV fistula for short.

As the name implies, an AV fistula connects an artery and a vein. The newly created vessel grows big and strong over time to allow the increased blood flow necessary to get the treatment done in a decent amount of time. Without the accelerated flow, dialysis patients would basically live on the machine.

Because of the huge blood flow, the fistula also gives off a buzz, or a "thrill" in dialysis lingo. If you have someone feel the buzz in your arm, they're guaranteed to look at you like you're some kind of space alien.

But it's a great entertainment piece at parties.

The fistula takes time to "mature" after the surgery. So while it's maturing, they use the catheter for your dialysis treatments.

Once the fistula matures, or becomes big enough to support the blood flow needed, on come the needles.

Ongoing dialysis treatments involve inserting two fifteen-gauge (quite large) needles into the fistula. One needle takes the blood out of your system to process through the artificial kidney, and the other returns the cleaned blood back into the body.

The process would make a vampire salivate.

As my fistula was still in the process of maturing, I could sense that the attendants in my dialysis center were chomping at the bit to get a crack at it. The attendants or nurse would eventually have the responsibility of inserting the needles once the fistula was being used.

While I was still being dialyzed through the catheter, the attendants would walk by my chair, look down at my arm, and smile. One attendant even made the comment, "My, that's a juicy one."

I didn't know whether to laugh or yell for help.

I had visions of the attendants chasing me down the hall with a needle in each hand yelling, "Don't worry, this won't hurt a bit!"

Once they started using my fistula and needles, I learned real fast that some attendants are better "stickers" than others. Some can insert needles with minimal pain, while others were probably Gestapo in a previous life.

Once the needles go in your arm, the treatment is underway. Again, each treatment is three to four hours, so there is a lot of time to kill.

The best advice I can give patients having to go through this is to find something to do to make the time pass quickly.

Some lucky souls can actually sleep while being treated, but that is something I've never been able to do. Others will watch the chairside TV.

Reading is my number one pastime. I bought an iPad, which, in addition to being an electronic reader, allows me to stay current on my email and surf the web while on dialysis.

The treatment itself can sometimes go off without a hitch. But, there also may be frequent complications, including dizziness, cramping, pain, nausea, vomiting, fainting, itching, and a generally poor attitude toward the whole process.

Now, it would be unusual to have all these side effects in the same treatment, but unfortunately, not impossible.

Yet there is a lot you can do in between treatments to minimize the chances of any (or all) of these taking place.

For instance, the less fluid you gain in between treatments, the lower your chance of cramping. Cramping is generally caused by the machine removing too much fluid too fast.

My goal to have the best possible dialysis treatment with the fewest side effects is a driver of my philosophy of abstention from the things that are supposed to be limited. Even small portions of foods high in sodium, potassium, and/or phosphorous can affect a dialysis patient's long-term health and make the treatment more miserable than it already is.

Know Your Stuff

The dialysis machine is really a scientific marvel, and it's important for dialysis patients to understand as much about their treatments as possible.

The importance of learning about my treatment became clear to me early on when some doctor who I had never seen before came up to me during a treatment and said that my albumin was too low.

With seven years of advanced education and thirty years in industry, the most brilliant response I could come up with was "Huh?"

Turns out, albumin is a measure of my protein intake. When your kidneys are failing, you're supposed to limit the amount of protein you take in. But once you start dialysis, you're supposed to *increase* your protein because the treatments weaken you so much.

Understanding that helped improve my quality of life.

So, one of my guiding principles of living with dialysis is knowing my stuff.

It's a lesson I learned early in my business career.

I was a young analyst at a big company. The vice president in charge of my area was making an unannounced tour through my department.

He was a serious type and very dour in his approach. He had no hint of a sense of humor.

Then my colleagues and I realized, to our horror, that he was grilling people and asking associates detailed questions as part of his tour.

We strongly considered asking for early retirement or cutting through the red tape and just running screaming from the building.

But, we stayed put and when he got to me, he barked, "Do you know your division's profit goals?"

I had a wild impulse to say, "No, but if you hum a few bars…"

But, with that thought of professional suicide contained, I rattled off some numbers that were close enough that he didn't suggest that I find another line of work.

Before he left my department, he leaned over and said, "Good, if you know 'em, it's easier to make 'em."

I think the old coot was onto something.

Similarly, knowing about the technical aspects of your dialysis treatment will benefit your health in the long run.

Of course knowing what to do and what not to do takes time. Living with kidney failure and being treated through dialysis is a balancing act.

The artificial kidney cleans your blood indiscriminately, which means that some beneficial elements get filtered out as well. So, dialysis patients have to take in enough to counteract the filtration process, but not so much that they raise the undesirable readings to harmful levels.

A patient has to become an expert in the blood test readings and the specifics of the treatment to keep this balance in place.

Keep Your Balance

Getting back to the treatment, your vital signs are monitored throughout the marathon dialysis session.

While on dialysis, it can get really interesting to watch your blood pressure, a measure that is very much in your best interest to keep steady. And low.

As I mentioned earlier, one of the effects of gaining too much fluid in between treatments is elevated blood pressure, which is never a good thing.

So, as your machine is syphoning off the excess fluid, you could be watching your pressure heading in the same direction as profits in the automotive industry.

In one single treatment, you can go from feeling uptight because your BP is too high to feeling mellow as it comes down to normal levels to feeling dizzy and crampy as it keeps declining and to fainting dead out in your chair as it gets too low.

Then, the attendant or nurse will have to add some fluid in the form of saline solution to your bloodstream to get the pressure back up to the normal range again.

Like I said, it's a balancing act.

Come Here Often?

There's definitely a sense of camaraderie amongst dialysis patients.

My current center has twelve chairs, although I've seen places with as many as forty chairs. These chairs are all closely placed in one very large treatment room.

So, you're in close proximity to your neighbors, and seeing as you go there three times a week and stay for between four and five hours each time, you see a lot of your fellow patients.

In addition, you have a once-a-week consult with your doctor during your treatment, all within earshot of everybody else, so we patients have few secrets from each other.

The doctors want to be sure you're following your regimen. They know *everything* about you from the battery of blood tests taken every other week. Most doctors will really get on your case if any of your readings are out of whack, and they are always quick to assume it is because you are straying from your diet.

One time, a guy sitting next to me was getting grilled about his diet. His phosphorous level was over 11.0 (normal is between 3.0 and 5.5.) His other key readings were not so great either.

The patient was trying to slough it off, claiming that the readings were bad and that he wasn't doing anything wrong, etc., etc.

But it was his worst nightmare. The doctor and nurse were asking questions, and his girlfriend was present to correct his not-so-true answers.

The conversation went something like this:

Phosphorous high:

Patient: "Can't imagine why, try to watch my intake, religiously take my binders."

Girlfriend: "You drink milk with every meal and snack. We went out to eat three times this week; you skipped your binders each time. You eat peanut butter cookies like there's a shortage, and last night you scarfed down half a bag of peanuts and washed it down with a cold beer."

Potassium high:

Patient: "Not sure why. Followed my diet to the letter."

Girlfriend: "We went out for Italian on Saturday. You had spaghetti and meatballs with extra tomato sauce. You think pizza is a health food. And, you think you can eat all the potatoes you want as long as they're deep fried to wash away all the bad stuff."

Fluid overload:

Patient: "Think my dry weight needs to be adjusted."

Girlfriend: "You might think about not guzzling through a garden hose, swishing down Coke and beer. And my milk budget is on the level of bank bailout funds."

The patient was actually glad I was in the chair next to him, and he looked to me for moral support. With each girlfriend revelation, he would just turn to me and shrug his shoulders as if to say, "What can you do?" And then we would just laugh. But obviously, the issues were very serious to his short-term and long-term health, so he had to make some lifestyle changes to get his levels back in line.

If a dialysis patient ever needs the equivalent of group therapy, there is never a shortage of sympathetic ears at a dialysis center. You need look no further than your nearest neighbor to your left or right to find someone facing many of the same challenges as you're confronting day in and day out.

The Traveling Circus

One of the great challenges of being on dialysis is traveling.

If you're going away for any length of time, you have to make arrangements to have dialysis treatments at a center close to where you're staying.

Unfortunately, it's never as easy as just calling and telling the other center when you'll be showing up. You have to be sure they have room for you and that you can get your treatment on your regular treatment day and at your requested time.

I always prefer to have my treatments first thing in the morning. Of course, while I was working full time, this wasn't possible, but when I was traveling for vacation, I would always request mornings, or "first shift" in dialysis center lingo.

When I was traveling, I always had to hope and pray that the remote center could start my treatment on the day and hour that I wanted. If not, and if my begging and pleading were ineffective, I had to either start at another time later in the day or look for another center likely to be even farther away from wherever I was staying.

Once you have the schedule and place that you want, your existing center has to transmit copies of your medical records, including your most recent test results, to the new center.

If your tuberculosis test isn't current, you'll have to get another one before the other center will let you in. The test involves your center's nurse sticking yet another needle under your skin, ignoring your yelp of pain, and injecting you with test fluid. If you come back in another couple of days and the site doesn't look like a small rodent burrowed up under your epidermis, you're clear to go.

I found out what traveling while on dialysis was like soon after I started needing treatments.

My wife was going to Arizona to compete in a tennis tournament, and after much discussion, we decided that I would go with her.

As an aside, if you're ever looking for a place where it would be easy to keep your fluid gain under control, Arizona is for you.

The average humidity is about zero percent, and after playing a little tennis, with my fluid restriction and all, I felt like someone could have rolled me up and put me on one of those storage hooks in the garage.

Anyway, as I was coming up on the appointment time of my remote treatment, I was feeling a little trepidation (read: fear) about going someplace other than my usual center.

I started thinking about the quality (and attitude) of the attendants and nurses, along with the cleanliness and setup of the center. Who's going to put my needles in?!?

I can now tell you from experience that there's a wide variance in these factors from center to center.

So, first I had to find the place, which was no small task. The center was buried behind a hotel and a shopping strip center.

I walked in, and my first impression was okay; the place seemed clean and well-staffed.

But, I was still a little uncomfortable, and my discomfort usually manifests itself as feeble attempts at humor.

A lady, who I guessed was the charge nurse, came up to me and said, "Are you looking for a chair?"

I said, "Yes, and a dialysis treatment would be nice, too, ha ha ha ha…"

She just looked at me completely straight-faced.

I stopped my little laugh with an <ahem>.

She looked at her schedule and said, "Are you Robert?"

I said, "Yes, but please call me Bob. The last time I was called Robert, I was caught red-handed looking at bikinibabes.com, ha ha ha ha…"

Nothing. Not even a twitch.

<Ahem>

I could see that my attempt at humor was going nowhere, so I just shut up and got on with the treatment, which went pretty well overall.

It doesn't take long once you start these treatments to discover that you want your needles inserted a certain way and you want some other things done just so. Once you move to another center, even temporarily, your comfort zone with your usual nurses and attendants goes out the window.

I explained my particular desires to my attendant in Arizona and after what I perceived as a bit of an "Are you for real?" look, she complied pretty nicely.

The bottom line is that you *can* travel while you're on dialysis, but it takes a little extra planning. And lots of courage.

Sometimes It Works...Sometimes It Doesn't

I can think of two of my early treatments that represent a kind of microcosm of how well (or poorly) each session can go.

One was very early in my dialysis life before they were even using my fistula—as in, no painful sticks, and other potential complications that arise with the use of needles, including being scared out of your wits when the attendants come at you with them.

So the old catheter was still being used.

Now, when my kidneys were failing and before starting dialysis, I was pretty sick. And, say what you will about these treatments, they really make you feel a lot better.

Your blood is being filtered properly, and your fluid is kept in balance, although finding the right "dry weight," can be somewhat trial and error at first. (Your dry weight is your post-treatment body weight target. They use it to determine how much fluid to remove during each treatment.)

Anyway, this early treatment was going very well. I had no sticks, no complications, felt pretty good, and brought plenty of things to do during my three-and-a-half hours that made the time go by relatively quickly.

So, I was in a good mood when the treatment was coming to a close, joking with all the attendants. And, when I was done, I popped up out of my chair, ready to go home. This was the way treatment was supposed to work, and I was the original ninja dialysis patient.

The other example that was completely contrary to this la-de-da, happy, peppy session happened *after* they started using my fistula.

Remember the surgically-altered vessel carrying five times the normal blood volume? With needles?

The fistula goes the length of my forearm, and the attendants are supposed to move the needle sticks up and down the arm in different places so as not to wear out any one place or let excessive scar tissue develop in any one area.

And, keep in mind, the quality of needle sticks varies widely from sticker to sticker.

On this particular day, my attendant was one who I considered to be a "good sticker." She could usually put those gigantic needles in with minimal discomfort.

However, keeping with the process of moving the needles up and down the arm, the attendant was going to try an area further up on my arm that had not been used before.

So, the "bottom" needle was inserted just fine, and it was positioned in an area that had been used before.

The "upper" needle hurt a little more than normal going in. But, I didn't think much of it since it was inserted in a new area. I just sucked it up and didn't say anything.

After the treatment was started, I looked down at my arm, and everything seemed normal, so I just started reading my book.

After a few minutes, though, I looked again and thought that my arm was starting to look a little abnormal. But, still considering myself a dialysis rookie, and basically being too dumb to know any better, I didn't say anything and just went on reading.

A little while later, I looked down again and had to stop myself from having a coronary.

My forearm looked like grandma's Thanksgiving gourd on industrial strength Miracle-Grow.

The first words I was able to utter were something reactionary like "Holy crap."

Then, still not very sure of myself, I tried to stay calm, forced a smile, and signaled to one of the attendants.

"Um…excuse me, but it seems like something isn't one hundred percent right here…"

She immediately hightailed it over to my chair saying, "What's going on?" along the way.

I said, "Well, if my arm gets any bigger we're going to be able to enter it in the Macy's Thanksgiving Day Parade."

This woman was a hardened veteran dialysis attendant, but when she saw my arm, even her eyes grew wide.

"Holy crap," she said.

My sentiments exactly.

Turns out, I learned my first lesson on "infiltration." In that hugely unfortunate set of circumstances, the needle actually goes right through the fistula vessel, causing your return blood, dialysate fluid, saline, and just about everything short of the kitchen sink to go right into the tissue under your skin, instead of traveling along its merry way into your bloodstream where it belongs.

Infiltration can be fairly common with newly formed fistulas that aren't yet completely mature—or, in my case, when your sticker is trying a new area on the vessel, as they're supposed to.

So, this particular infiltration was pretty much a crisis situation. They had to stop the treatment; otherwise, the equivalent of the Missouri River was going to continue flowing into my arm.

They didn't want to pull the needles out right away, so they brought me some ice to try to bring the swelling down. I sat there for a while with my ice, attempting to quell the urge to go into complete panic mode.

After what seemed like an eternity, but in reality was only a few minutes, the attendant and nurse came over to assess whether they could re-stick the needle in another area and continue my treatment.

You might be thinking, well, why didn't they just call it a day and send you home—kind of like the ironic equivalent of calling in sick from dialysis.

Well, rescheduling treatment is only done under the most extreme of circumstances. Generally, it's not advisable to miss or shorten *any* dialysis treatment. Remember, substituting ongoing, twenty-four-hour-per-day, seven-days-per-week kidney function with three four-hour treatments per week to keep all your critical readings balanced is a dicey proposition at best.

Not having your full treatment when you're supposed to can truly have dire consequences.

Yes, I'll say it—up to and including death.

Now, it's not likely that you'll kick the old bucket from missing one treatment. But it is possible, and, let's face it, if it happens, you don't get a do-over. You can't just say, "Okay, I get it now. I'll do better next time." It's over, buddy; the curtain is closed.

Now, if they want to re-stick and continue your treatment after infiltrating, the new site has to be *above* the infiltration spot or further up on your arm. If the needle insertion were to occur below the infiltration site, the fluid and all its buddies would just continue pouring through the new, unintentional hole in your vessel once the machine was turned back on.

Right at this particular time, however, re-sticking me above the infiltration point was really not an option. That area was so swollen that the needle would have to have been like a foot long to even get to the fistula.

So, discretion being the better part of valor and all, it was decided that I would be sent home. The nurse told me to keep the ice on my arm overnight and come back the next day for another try, which I agreed to do.

Mind you, this wasn't as simple a decision as it seemed for a couple of reasons.

For one, this all happened on a Wednesday—part of my normal treatment sequence of Monday, Wednesday, and Friday.

So having to come in again on Thursday meant that I would get stuck for three consecutive days—a thought that didn't exactly make me want to jump for joy. In addition, I had carefully aligned my meeting schedule at work to leave a little earlier than normal on Monday, Wednesday, and Friday. This, in turn, meant that I had late meetings on Thursday, which would have to be rescheduled.

But, under the circumstances, leaving and coming back the next day seemed like the least wrong decision to make.

So, as a contrast to that early session with the catheter when I sprang up out of the chair after treatment and was the real life of the party, this time I was somewhat demoralized. I got up, looking like Popeye on steroids with my arm swollen to ridiculous proportions, and kind of slunk out of the center, muttering, "See you tomorrow."

Later that evening watching me attempt to eat would have been comical if it weren't so painful.

I scooped up a fork full of vegetables and was bringing it up to my mouth when the bending of my arm hit the swelling point and stopped the fork mid-journey, causing the veggies to fly off the fork and spill all over my lap.

The wife was just looking at me, but I could tell she was trying not to laugh.

So, I just said, "Hmm. Wonder what it's like to eat left-handed."

And we both started to laugh.

Those two treatments typify life on dialysis. Some treatments go without a hitch, and some render you practically incapacitated afterward.

After some treatments, it's like the first example—you feel great and you're ready to spring into action after sitting for such a long time.

After others, it's all you can do to make it out of the center on your own two feet.

That's Not All...(Other Complications)

Bleeding

It may seem like stating the obvious, since, after all, dialysis entails your entire blood supply running through plastic tubes, being cleansed, and then rolling back into your body, but one of the most common risks of being on dialysis is...well... bleeding.

In addition to the infiltration noted previously, post-treatment bleeding can also be an issue. When the garden-hose-sized needles are removed, pressure needs to be applied to the needle sites. This is done either with your free hand or with plastic clamps.

The amount of time you need to maintain the pressure is far from being an exact science. And, remember the accelerated blood flow. When patients are applying pressure to these needle sites, we're not just keeping the sites from bleeding. We're keeping them from *gushing*.

Even after you, the nurse, and the attendant have all agreed that the bleeding has stopped for good, the sites are all bandaged up, and you think you're good to go, there's still a chance that one or both sites could let go, and it's Niagara Falls all over again.

It's like, "Cleanup in aisle six."

Dialysis is truly not for the squeamish. Fact is, if you are squeamish, you won't be for long once you start dialysis.

Among some of the other pleasures that visit us with some regularity:

Cramping

A dialysis staple.

Cramping is caused by the machine removing fluid from the body faster than your kidneys would normally do it. This accelerated removal rate can sometimes cause your muscles to tighten up.

Again, it doesn't happen all the time, and sometimes it can surprise you.

Early on, in my clueless stage, I wasn't really attuned to the possibility of cramping. I found out about it shortly after starting on dialysis.

I was finished with my treatment and all excited about making a quick escape from the center. My attendant was making conversation while I was still seated. I got up from my chair as he was still talking to me. He turned around to put some equipment away, and when he turned back around toward me, I was gone.

Turns out, when I stood up my leg muscles cramped and down I went. The attendant was surprised because he wasn't really expecting to continue his conversation with me lying on the floor.

When you cramp that bad, the only cure is to walk around to loosen your muscles up again. Of course, when it's really bad, you have to have attendants half-carry you while you try to get the feeling back in your legs.

Cramps can also sneak up on you well after your treatment is over.

When I was doing my treatment in the evening, it wasn't unusual for cramps to hit when I was in bed several hours after the session ended.

I could be sound asleep in bed one minute and up hopping around like a cartoon character—"Oooooh, I hurt my little leg…"—the next.

Sometimes cramps can even hit the next day. While you're at work. In a meeting.

Basically, cramps are like lightning. They can strike anytime, anywhere and without warning.

The easiest way to *prevent* cramping is to limit your fluid gain between treatments. The more fluid the machine has to take off, the more likely you are to cramp.

In extreme circumstances, like if you're cramped so bad the attendants have to ball you up and roll you out to your car, they will give you something salty to drink, like chicken broth, before you leave.

The salt causes fluid to be absorbed into your muscles, which will ease the cramping. Attendants can also add saline to your treatment mix if you cramp *during* the treatment, which is truly not a lot of fun.

Using broth to counter cramps should be done with caution, however. As we'll discuss later, anything salty will make you thirsty, which might cause you to gain even more fluid and make your *next* treatment a challenge.

So, there can be a cyclical pattern between cramping, sodium intake, and fluid balance.

There's no rest for the weary on dialysis.

Dizziness/Fainting

Dizziness and fainting are generally caused by a drop in your blood pressure. A drop in blood pressure is a close relative of cramping, as both can be symptoms of the machine removing too much fluid. In addition to causing your muscles to seize, this can cause your blood pressure to drop at an accelerated rate. Low blood pressure can cause dizziness or even fainting.

Low blood pressure needs to be monitored even after your treatment is complete, especially if you take medications to keep your BP regulated on an ongoing basis.

Doctors will generally advise you not to take your BP pills before treatment, as they don't want the machine to filter the medicine out of your bloodstream.

After I first started dialysis, I was getting my treatments in the evening and then going home and taking my BP pills.

The treatment was effectively bringing my pressure down, and then taking the pills was bringing it down even further. This would sometimes bring on the dizziness/fainting episodes.

My wife would know I was fuzzing out if I started talking nonsense.

She'd be talking to me normally, something like:

My wife: "So, you about ready to turn in?"

Me: "Yeah, but first, we better pull the hiking boots out of the trees."

When I said something like that, she would know that either my senility was getting worse or that I was dizzy from low blood pressure.

Or both.

Not to be repetitive, but controlling your fluid intake is the best way to avoid getting dizzy or fainting outright (which I've also experienced) due to blood pressure getting low.

You may also want to consult with your doctor about blood pressure thresholds under which you might adjust your medication dosage, especially after treatments.

Nausea/Vomiting

No real explanation is needed here. Treatments can readily induce both of these lovely side effects.

Everybody's different, but I've never wanted to eat within a two-hour window before my treatment started. Just through experience, I found that if I did, enough nausea to light up Times Square was pretty much a sure thing.

In addition, I learned that the digestive process draws blood toward the stomach, which could bring on the previously mentioned cramping and/or dizziness/fainting. So, I've always wanted to start my treatment with an empty stomach.

Now, opinions will vary widely on this issue, and eating and drinking while on treatment is actually quite common.

I even had one patient near me who ordered a pizza from her cell phone while she was being dialyzed.

I was like, okay, where should we start? With the fact that she's eating pizza, which is the poster child for diet no-no's in the dialysis world? Or with the fact that she's not only eating, but eating heavily while on her treatment?

You might be wondering why the dialysis attendants would allow a patient to do this. I have to defend them somewhat; they're in a difficult position between fulfilling their responsibility to ensure that each patient is getting a good treatment and telling an adult what he or she should or shouldn't be doing.

I've seen very different approaches regarding accountability issues like this in the different centers that I've been to.

From my perspective, it's a no-brainer…no eating or drinking while I'm being treated—or shortly before being treated.

Needless to say, having to sit relatively still for a four-hour treatment is bad enough, but having to do it with an upset stomach is setting new standards for miserable.

Itching

This is probably the least serious yet *most* aggravating potential side effect of dialysis.

There are two potential causes of dialysis-related itching.

First, and most serious, is the possibility that the phosphorous levels in the blood are too high—something that should be evident from the frequent blood tests that are taken. Itching is a symptom of high phosphorous.

Second, if, like me, you have dry skin to begin with, the dialysis process can dry your skin even further through the removal of fluid from your system.

As with everything else, I learned this lesson the hard way when I first started on dialysis.

I didn't know how important it was to watch my phosphorous intake, and I was pretty hit-or-miss on taking my binders with meals.

In addition, it was wintertime, and, as I mentioned, my skin was pretty dry and itchy to begin with.

So, I would get these bouts of itching, causing me to scratch multiple places at the same time. I looked like I was doing a cross between the Macarena and an Irish jig.

The strange thing was when I was talking to someone and scratching constantly, the other person would start having imaginary itches, and pretty soon they would be scratching too.

You don't think of itching as being infectious, but, trust me, I know otherwise.

Again, I'm not really a great person to provide a solution, since I was the one doing everything short of rolling on the front lawn to get to some of my itches. All I can do is tell you what has worked for me.

First and foremost, watch your phosphorous intake and take your binders. As discussed, high phosphorous can have a wide range of very serious long-term consequences as well.

Once I started controlling my diet and found religion on taking my binders, much of the itching subsided.

As far as the dry skin goes, I've found that using a moisturizer, especially right after showering and during cold weather can help. This helped me before I even knew what dialysis was.

I don't mean to portray these side effects as being mutually exclusive.

I've had treatments where multiple combinations have all hit at the same time. What fun that is.

And, of course, these are all really secondary complications.

The primary problem with not dialyzing properly is much more serious.

And permanent.

So, the best things patients can do for themselves—all of which are fundamental for dialysis patients—include the following:

- Never miss a treatment. Stay for the entire process wherever possible. Even asking to be taken off treatment a few minutes early can have consequences.

- Follow the dietary guidelines and take your binders.

- Manage your fluid intake. Try to avoid putting on too much in between treatments.

Lifestyle

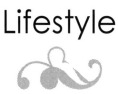

Imagine you're just moseying along minding your own business.

Life is good.

You feel great. You are free to go anywhere you want. No restrictions.

On a whim, you decide that since there's nothing going on, you think you'll up and go to Vegas where you will eat what you want, drink what you want, stay up all night—whatever.

Then you hear this voice that says, "Oh, say pal, about those freedoms?"

You say, warily, "Yeah, what about them?"

Buzzzz. "Not so much anymore."

You'd be like, "Well, what exactly do you mean?"

The voice says, "Going anywhere you want on a whim? That's out."

"Huh?"

"Oh, you can still hit Vegas, but we'll need one month's notice. And, of course, you'll need to call in advance to make sure everything's okay with your appointment."

"Well, okay, I guess I can do that."

"Oh, and you might not be able to get the schedule that you want; you'll have to work around availability."

"You mean Vegas might not be available?"

"Exactly."

So, this rocks your foundation a little bit, but it still seems workable.

Then, you start imagining the details.

"Can't wait to hit my favorite Italian place. Think I'll start with some *prosciutto*, or maybe some *minestrone* soup."

That voice again.

Buzzzz.

"Prosciutto has about a week's worth of sodium. And, if you have that minestrone, between the sodium and the fluid, you'll bloat up like the federal budget deficit."

You start thinking, "Geez, that kind of sucks."

Then you think, "Well, okay. We'll skip the appetizers and go right to the great main course. Think I'll dive into some linguine with extra-meat tomato sauce or maybe some lasagna."

Buzzzz.

You think, "Now what?"

"Sure, have whatever dish you want, but without tomato sauce, or any tomato-based product," says the voice.

"In an Italian restaurant? That'll leave me with a salad and a meatball."

"Uh, just make sure there's no funny seasoning in that meatball."

You think, "Oh boy, this sure is taking the fun out of this dinner."

"All right, well, this is my decadent weekend; I'll skip dinner and go right to the dessert. I know a place that has a chocolate *sformato* that's to die for. It's a cake filled with chocolate pudding with almonds on top and Amaretto whipped cream."

Buzzzz.

"No chocolate. Or almonds. And whipped cream? Forget it."

You start feeling frustrated.

"All right. Like I said. Decadent, right? Forget about eating. I'm in Vegas. I'll get all my calories from booze. Heh heh. Party the night away."

The voice is like, "Well…."

"What now?"

"You can have a drink, but don't go overboard. You can only have so much fluid per day, and alcohol can raise your blood pressure."

"So much fluid per day? That doesn't include the coffee that I sip all day long, right? And the eight glasses of water and all that?"

"Well, yes, all fluid is included as well as Jello, ice cream, and anything that's liquid at room temperature."

"Yikes."

"Oh, and as far as staying out all night, just remember your set schedule."

"What?"

"Yeah, your days of running around free and easy?"

"Yeah?"

Buzzzz.

"Oh boy."

"Yeah, you're going to have to be sure you work around a roughly five-hour period where you're going to be in one set place and sit still the whole time."

"Think I'll pass."

"Oh, it's not a matter of choice."

"What if I decide to just not show up?"

"Then you might be visiting that great casino in the sky."

"Pardon?"

"Yep, as in the big sayonara."

"All right, well I'll go, but I'll just have fun the rest of my time there."

"Well…."

"What? I won't have fun?"

"Well, that five hours I mentioned?"

"Yeah…"

"Well, it might drain you of all your strength and make you feel like crap the rest of the time."

"Why, what are they going to do?"

"Well, they're going to put two really big needles in your arm, draw out all your blood, run it through a machine, and then put it back."

"Like hell they are."

"Oh yeah, remember, your alternative is to roll dice with old Gabriel up there near the big pearly gates."

"Geez."

"Oh, and in addition, during this treatment you might have some minor discomfort."

"How minor?"

"Well, there's the pain of those needles, and you might have some dizziness, bleeding, muscle cramps, itching, restlessness, and heart palpitations. Oh, and there's always a possibility you could blow chunks."

"Holy moly."

The voice goes on.

"But, hey, don't you fret none, just go ahead on your trip and have a good old time."

You think for a minute, then you say, "How?"

The rest of this section includes a discussion of some of the areas where being on dialysis affects your lifestyle.

Truth be told, there aren't many parts of your lifestyle that are left unaffected.

Eating

I've already touched on the dietary restrictions faced by dialysis patients, but when you have to start paying attention to the ingredients in everything you eat, you start to realize how pervasive these dietary no-no's are in everyday food choices.

Sometimes it feels like you're on a bread-and-water diet.

(Oh, but no whole wheat bread, and watch the amount of water.)

And, again, it's not like if you misbehave, your biggest risk is splitting the seams on your favorite trousers.

There are serious long-term health problems associated with not following the dialysis diet.

Eating out in restaurants can present its own challenges.

When the implications of my new dietary restrictions first started to sink in, I have to admit, it flipped me out a little bit.

My wife and I planned to go out to a restaurant shortly after I began dialysis, the first time we had been out in a while because I had been so sick. It was also the first chance for me to see how hard it was going to be to order something off a menu within the constraints of this new diet.

Now, I should mention that even before getting sick I had a tendency to misbehave in public outings. My wife was always a little leery of going out because the potential for embarrassment was high.

So this first time going out since starting dialysis was no different. She cautioned me against pulling any of my airhead pranks on the waiter.

But, as I was going through the menu, it seemed like every selection had something in it that I wasn't supposed to eat.

I was feeling a combination of frustration and being pissed off at my set of circumstances.

So, when the waiter came over, I acted all proper and said, "Yes, I'd like an appetizer of nachos with no chips, cheese, or salsa."

The poor guy looked confused, but I went on.

"A side salad with no tomatoes, cheese, or dressing. Oh, and light on the lettuce." I leaned over and said knowingly to my wife on the side, "A lot of water content in lettuce, you know." <wink wink>

The waiter had stopped writing and was just staring at me, stunned. The wife was just rolling her eyes.

"And for the entrée, a pepperoni pizza with no sauce, cheese, or pepperoni."

"Y-y-y-yes sir, anything else?"

I said, "Oh yeah, for my drink, I'd like water…but go easy on the fluid."

So, the waiter went on his way and my wife tried to find a graceful way to crawl under the table.

The experience gave me a sense of what I was in for in terms of dining out.

Eating in any uncontrolled environment can be a challenge. If you are going out to a restaurant, it is a good idea to look at menus online before choosing where to go.

Some online menus will even provide the content of dishes in terms of fat, sodium, and carbohydrates.

Sometimes, however, there are circumstances beyond your control like going to someone's house for dinner. In those instances, all you can do is work around the things that are really off-limits and have small portions of other foods that might be questionable.

You have to do all this without making your hostess think that her cooking sucks or that you secretly think she's a serial killer trying to poison her guests.

Dialysis is funky because the filtration system is *dumb*. It takes some valuable nutrients out of your system at the same time that it removes impurities.

The net effect of this dumb filtration system is that your body tends to crave calorie input at the same time you are faced with these onerous dietary restrictions. The dietician in the dialysis center will want to make sure that you're eating well enough to make up this calorie deficit.

And, of course you tend to get a hankering for many of the things you shouldn't have.

When my wife and I walk down an aisle in the grocery store with a lot of prepared foods, I practically have to roll my tongue up off the floor.

Hamburger Helper, Chunky Soup. Mmmmmmm.

And, don't even bring up Chef Boyardee.

Being on dialysis really magnifies these hankerings. Between craving calories and not being able to eat some of their favorite foods, dialysis patients can get a little crazy.

Call it the ***Hungry Horror*** syndrome.

In addition, the long treatments can upset the timing of your meals, which can make the Hungry Horrors even worse.

Getting hungry was particularly challenging when I was being dialyzed in the evening after work.

As I mentioned, I was never one to eat while being treated, as many of my shift mates would do.

In fact, I found that it really wasn't a good idea to eat within a couple of hours of starting the treatment either. If I did, I'd usually develop enough nausea to kill a small elephant.

So, on treatment days, I would have lunch around noon, and have nothing else to eat until after my treatment, usually around eight in the evening at the earliest.

The combination of not having eaten in a while and the machine depleting whatever useful nutrients that were left in my body made for a pretty dire situation hunger-wise.

On the way home, it took about every ounce of strength I had left to keep from raiding the local McDonald's.

I'd go crazy thinking about ordering up some ridiculous sandwich like a triple quarter-pounder with extra cheese and maybe a couple dozen chicken nuggets. Then maybe I could stop somewhere else and wash the whole thing down with a pepperoni pizza.

Of course, I wouldn't actually eat any of that stuff; I'd just think about it *really* hard.

By the time I actually got home, I'd want to eat up every ounce of dinner as well as the placemat, tablecloth, and even the plastic phony fruit, bowl and all.

Going to work the next day would be even worse. Around about ten in the morning, the Hungry Horrors would take over my life.

Heaven forbid someone at work should mention food in a routine conversation.

Once, I was in a sidebar discussion in a meeting, and one person said that someone she had disagreed with in the meeting was "dumb as a bowl of spaghetti."

I started thinking, hmmm, a bowl of spaghetti, huh?

So, I continued on with the meeting, but later, someone else said they wanted to "get down to the meat of the matter."

That set me off to a bowl of spaghetti with meat sauce.

And toward the end of the meeting, everyone agreed that it was beneficial for the two opposing sides to "break bread" on their differences.

Now, I'm suspecting a conspiracy.

By the end of the meeting, I probably looked like one of those guys from *Night of the Living Dead*—willing to eat anything in sight.

So, we patients have to deal with the fact that the dialysis process makes us like hungry dogs in a meat locker, while, at the same time, seriously restricting what we can eat—pretty conflicting dynamics.

There are many such conflicts involved with living and eating on dialysis.

Take protein intake, for instance.

In late stages of kidney failure, doctors will tell you to limit your protein intake, as excess protein can further damage the kidneys. Then, after you begin dialysis, they start telling you to *increase* your protein because, again, the process can filter protein out of your system along with impurities.

Sheesh.

But every once in a while, if you really behave yourself, your blood test readings will allow you a little flexibility in your diet.

And when you haven't had some of your favorite food or drinks for a while, having even a taste of them becomes a big moment in your life.

A while back, I was getting together with some family members I hadn't seen in a while, and when they asked what was new, I responded with embarrassing enthusiasm.

"I HAD A COKE LAST WEEK!"

They just looked at me like I should be sitting off in a corner somewhere mumbling to myself and counting my own fingers.

As a brief explanation for my nutzo behavior, cola drinks, my personal favorite, are high in phosphorous, and, therefore, should be consumed on a very limited basis by anyone on dialysis.

But, my most recent lab results had showed that my blood levels of phosphorous were actually *too low*, which in many ways is just as dangerous as being too high. So my dialysis dietician recommended having some high-phosphorous foods or drinks that weekend.

I could have kissed her right then and there—well, except for the fact that I was confined to my dialysis chair and she was standing up.

So, my wife and I went out for lunch that Saturday, and I ordered up a cheeseburger, which I also hadn't had in a while, and a Coke. My wife wondered how anyone could consume a whole meal with such a stupid grin on his face.

These seemingly minor opportunities can have a big impact when you live with the many restrictions of life on dialysis.

I'd be remiss in completing a section on eating without saying more about how helpful my wife has been in managing my diet.

In addition to being a great companion as I go through the rigors of dialysis, she has put her substantial cooking skills to work, finding new ways to deal with the very limited foods that I can eat with my many restrictions.

Her cooking talent is particularly important for me because I'm hopelessly inept as a cook. If I tried to cut vegetables real fast like I see them do on TV, I'd end up chopping my fingers off and probably wouldn't stop until I got to the elbow.

On the diet front, we also have to be careful that the wife's not shorting *herself* of some valuable nutrients. While I have to be sure of not taking in too much potassium, for example, she needs to be sure she gets some in the foods that she eats, especially because she's a competitive tennis player. Physical activity can cause a loss of potassium, so she has to take in some extra in her diet.

This means that sometimes we're eating different things at the same meal, which is yet another challenge.

So, many thanks to my wife, and for those of you who might be cooking for a dialysis patient, be sure to eat a balanced diet yourself. Add back important nutrients that are limited in the renal diet.

Drinking

Now when I say drinking, I'm specifically talking about fluids, not booze.

Forget about booze; I'm not addressing it here at all.

Well, okay, I'll talk about it later.

Anyway, fluid intake may be the most challenging dialysis-related limitation of them all.

Remember how taking in too much fluid between treatments can cause serious health issues, including the biggest one? And how excess fluid will make your next treatment a lot less pleasant?

It is a dialysis patient's reality that we have to limit the amount that we drink and that we're often walking around thirsty as all get out.

Fortunately, there are ways you can manage your thirst. None of them are easy, mind you, but they are necessary for a dialysis patient's long-term well-being. More on that later, however.

The reason fluid is an issue for dialysis patients is that the kidneys are not clearing fluid from our bodies the way normally functioning kidneys do.

Basically, this means (and, sorry, there's really no graceful way of putting this) most dialysis patients don't, well...pee.

That's right. We may be whizzes at maintaining this difficult lifestyle, but we don't actually whiz ourselves.

The fact that dialysis patients don't urinate makes it critical that we watch our fluid intake between dialysis treatments.

Some of the issues that could arise if we take in too much fluid are related to water buildup in our hearts and lungs.

In addition, the more fluid that has to be removed during your treatment, the more likely you are to experience side effects like cramping and cratering blood pressures.

To summarize, dialysis patients can't have as much to drink as healthy people, so patients in general are a bunch of seriously thirsty campers, and thirst can make you pretty crazy at times.

The wife and I are on a beach vacation.

These are not terribly "active" vacations, mind you. For the most part, we're sitting in our beach chairs reading and occasionally listening to our iPods.

Sitting down by the water on a glorious, sun-drenched day is our idea of heaven. So, we're at the beach this day.

Suddenly, this incredible woman walks by.

She's physically buffed, perfectly proportioned, and wearing a skimpy bikini. She's carrying an iced tea in a clear plastic cup with lots of ice and a thick slice of lemon.

I start to breathe a little heavier as she walks by, which gets my wife's attention, although in a distant way.

Then, I let a little growl out, and the Mrs. starts to notice a little more.

Suddenly, she sees the direction I'm looking and sees the girl.

But, not being the jealous type, the wife lets it go.

Then, I growl a little more and squirm a little in my chair, annoying the wife a little.

She checks back on me a few moments later and I continue to stare, but the wife still doesn't say anything.

Then, without even being fully aware, my passion takes over and I verbalize my heated desire. In a throaty voice I say, "Boy does that drink look good."

The wife just looks at me, shakes her head, and goes back to reading her book.

Fluid restrictions make dialysis patients do crazy things, and sometimes the rest of the world just can't understand it.

When my wife and I go grocery shopping, I make sure we walk down the drink aisle. I know I can't partake, but I just like to *see* the different drinks.

If anybody were to question me about it, I'd say, "Hey, do I give you a hard time about *your* fantasies?"

Sometimes, you might find yourself in a mall saying, "Pssst, hey kid, five dollars for your Slurpee…"

Or, you might be at a dinner and someone asks to have their water glass refilled, and you get a sudden urge to stab them through the heart with your salad fork.

Or, you're in a famous place, say a museum, and everyone around you is looking wondrously at the exhibits. Instead, you're checking out the water fountains in the hallway.

Or, you're in a meeting at work and someone rolls in a coffee urn. Later, while serious business issues are being discussed, you're wondering how much of a scene it would cause if you positioned yourself backward and upside down so you could pour the coffee directly down your throat.

When I do have a drink within my daily allotment, I have found that having something ice-cold is better at quenching thirst. There are obviously many cold drinks available, but, at the risk of sounding really boring, good old ice water has worked the best for me.

Thing is, when you do have that ice-cold drink in front of you, you don't want anybody messing with it.

One time, the wife and I were having dinner at home, and she suddenly said, "Can I have a sip of your water?" and reached over for it.

I shouted, "NO!" and snatched it away before she could get it.

She just sat there looking at me.

I was a little embarrassed by my rash reaction, but the best I could come up with was, "Well…hey, it's not like you were choking or anything."

She just shook her head again. Just like on the beach.

The real solution to thirst for a dialysis patient has to do with diet. I've found that to control being thirsty all the time and making everyone around you want to have you locked up, you have to control the sodium in your diet.

Sounds like a simple thing, right? Just take that old salt shaker off your table and put it up in the attic or something.

Unfortunately, like just about everything else about this illness and lifestyle, it's not that simple. Actually, very little of a person's sodium intake typically comes from the shaker.

As you look closely at the ingredients in different kinds of food, you discover that just about any kind of prepared food is going to contain a lot of sodium. For most people, this means eliminating or limiting some of your favorite things to eat, which is never a pleasant prospect.

If you are able to prepare your own foods or if you have someone else who does it, look for ways to limit the amount of sodium added. There are some pretty good low-sodium recipes available online.

If you have to buy prepared foods, be sure to check the sodium content and try to minimize your sodium intake.

Trust me. Controlling sodium is the best way to ensure that you don't end up wanting to drink up the bath water. Dialysis patients will benefit in so many ways.

I actually plan my sodium intake for each day. Sounds real exciting, huh?

If I know we're going to a restaurant or to someone's house for a meal late in the day, I'll keep my sodium intake very low early and try to be careful about what I eat in the "uncontrolled" situation.

As far as the amount of fluid to take in every day, generally, I plan to have one eight-ounce drink per meal. (Remember, this is just what works for me. Everyone is different.) The tough part of this regimen is not having anything in the interim. Before I started dialysis, I used to walk around with a big glass of ice water in the afternoon and evening.

Not any more.

If you plan to go out for lunch and want to have a little extra iced tea, make up for it by decreasing your fluid intake in the morning and/or evening. My personal preference is to have two cups of coffee in the morning. But, if I do that, I skip my drink at lunch. I'm not saying it's easy to wait until dinner for your next drink, but again, dealing with thirst is one of a dialysis patient's greatest challenges.

On the subject of drinking, we can't forget about alcohol.

Although, if you drink enough, it might make you forget.

Some dialysis patients continue to imbibe after starting dialysis, but when I started treatments, I quit completely and it made me want to jump for joy.

Then I realized that to actually jump for joy about anything, I have to have a few pops in me.

Houston, we have a problem.

This is yet another of the conflicts we face as dialysis patients. Drinking clearly isn't good for us, but for many of us it can help with the stress of being on dialysis. I'll admit that before getting sick, I used to like a beer on occasion.

Then, when I first started the Big D, I was in the hospital and some doctor was having a little sit-down with me, running through all the things I wasn't supposed to do—a list that was quite lengthy, as you know.

He eventually got around to beer and explained about it containing a lot of phosphorous and sodium and that it was tough on the fluid restrictions, yada, yada, yada.

I remember thinking, why not beat the Christmas rush and start hating this guy now. After considering the issue, however, I decided he was right and that it was best for me to quit.

Sometimes, missing drinking is more situational in nature.

One time, an associate in the office had a brochure for an Oktoberfest event that was going to be held in her hometown over the weekend. I was looking through the brochure and there were a bunch of events listed. One was a "fun run" (a contradiction in terms if I've ever heard one.) But she was the athletic type, so I asked if she was planning to participate.

"No."

"Oh, so are you going for the Bike Rally?" I asked.

"Huh, if I was going to ride a bike for any distance worth mentioning, they'd have to call it the Bike Ralph, since that's what I'd do."

"Well, how about the Polka Contest?"

"Nope, too much chance of injury to me or to anybody standing nearby."

I was still flipping through the brochure.

"Carnival Rides?"

"Uh-uh."

"So, what exactly are you doing at this Oktoberfest?"

"Drinking beer."

"Aha."

I'll admit, that used to be my kind of event.

I wasn't a rehab case or anything, but in my pre-dialysis life, if you were getting a bunch of people together with the primary intent of getting pickled, I was there.

But I knew going into the Big D that giving up alcohol entirely was the right decision. And, for the most part, I don't miss it at all. Among the many things I've given up from my favorite list of food and drinks, booze probably isn't even in the top five.

Some of my goofball friends will go to no end pointing out what I'm missing by adopting this point of view. But then again, as I reply to them, I don't get hangovers.

Of course, there are other fringe benefits to quitting drinking other than substantially improving your health and making your dialysis treatments much more bearable.

I mean, you're a lot less likely to appear naked in public. Ever again!

You won't try to go to sleep in a wastebasket, which can be painful.

You'll never again bet money that you can sing every song from Meat Loaf's *Bat Out of Hell* album from memory. (Try doing that *without* imbibing, by the way.)

Then, there's the money you'll save from not buying the booze anymore.

And the money you'll save from not damaging the ceiling in your living room after trying to hang upside down from your Waterford Crystal chandelier.

So, on the one hand, no group of people that I can think of deserves to tie one on more than dialysis patients with all the stress we go through.

But, truth be told, the best policy is abstention.

The decrease in fluid intake alone makes quitting worthwhile, not to mention the harmful ingredients in some drinks, including phosphorous and sodium.

Alcohol can also do a number on your blood pressure, which is often a problem for dialysis patients.

And, it makes it more difficult to keep your body weight under control, which again, leads to a host of complications.

To summarize this section, I strongly recommend that dialysis patients do everything possible to keep their fluid intake under control.

One of the best things a patient can do is reduce their sodium intake. This will help keep the thirsty horrors under control.

And, as far as our old buddy booze goes, it's better to completely abstain, but if you have to drink, do so in moderation.

Exercise

Yet another of the many conflicts faced by dialysis patients is the need for exercise.

Working out and being on dialysis is not exactly a natural mix simply because most of the time you feel like crap.

After most treatments, a dialysis patient's idea of a vigorous workout is walking to the scale without falling down.

And yet, because dialysis does such a total number on us, both physically and mentally, we need to stay active as much as, if not more than, normal, healthy people.

Well, I'm here to tell you that while being on dialysis is not exactly conducive to a good exercise routine, it also doesn't preclude it.

Before getting sick, I was what could be called a workout fiend. I loved going to the gym and did a rigorous combination of cardio and resistance training. I was a good athlete in my younger years as I played multiple sports. As I got older, I saw exercise as a way of recapturing my youth.

Of course, when I first went on dialysis, one of my first thoughts was "Well, that blows any chance I had of being on the cover of *Muscle & Fitness* magazine." The way I felt at the time, I was more likely to be on the cover of *Sickly & Hopeless*.

The first consideration for a new dialysis patient is that starting or restarting an exercise routine takes time. You shouldn't expect to go back to your normal level of activity immediately after you start your treatments.

(As with everything else, you should check with your doctor before starting any new exercise routine or increasing physical activity.)

Starting to exercise is obviously a big adjustment after a dialysis patient begins treatments. You generally feel pretty weak, and thinking about exercise is not exactly a top priority.

I speak from experience here.

After starting the Big D, I gave it a couple of weeks and then thought, okay, I'm back in the game now, time to get back to my exercise routine!

So, there I was, a new dialysis patient, waltzing back into the gym without a clue about what was ahead of me.

I was working with a personal trainer at the time, and he always had me stretch on some mats at the back of the gym and then had me do a little "warm-up run" on the treadmill. So, my first time back, we got right back to that routine.

My trainer was big on encouraging words that were intended to make me work harder: **"C'mon Bob, couple more here, you got it, looking good"**—that kind of thing.

(The **stars** are meant to bring across the cheery, upbeat manner with which these phrases were delivered.)

I would always feel compelled to complete the interaction.

"Yep, feeling good here, got it going", etc. etc.

My first time back, the stretching went fine. The joints were a little stiff, but no major problems.

Then he said, "Okay, let's hit the treadmill for our warm-up run."

I was like, **"Right-o, I'm up for it."**

So, I started on the treadmill, and my trainer turned around to talk to someone else for a bit.

When he turned back toward me, I was lying flat on my back stretched out on the warm-up mats.

If you looked at me from above, I was splayed out like da Vinci's Vitruvian Man.

At first, my trainer was stunned speechless, just staring at me.

Finally, he found his voice and was like, "Bob, what gives?"

In my stupor, I just kept on with my usual banter, **"No problem, just catching my breath here. Gonna get right back to it."** But I still lay motionless.

That positive reinforcement was so hard-wired into me that they could have been carting me off on a stretcher, and I still would have been saying things like, **"Little setback here, no big deal, see you soon…"**

My trainer didn't know exactly what to do, but after repeated failed attempts on my part to get up off the mat, he was about ready to call in the EMTs.

I think it was safe to say that I tried to do a little too much, too soon.

So, after temporarily giving up on the full-blown gym routine, I figured I would start slow with some other exercise and work my way up.

My wife and I figured we would walk the neighborhood. Walking is great exercise, and you can go at your own pace.

Now, you have to understand that my wife is a top-notch tennis player. She's in great shape. And, we're both competitive people by nature. But she was more than happy to walk with me.

Of course, our walks presented their own challenges.

By nature of her playing tennis regularly, and me just having been sick, she was in much better shape than I was when we started walking.

Although we agreed that our walks would be at a leisurely pace, our natural competitiveness took over at times, and we found ourselves going faster, silently challenging each other to keep up.

And, of course, I was too stubborn and proud to beg illness and ask her to slow down.

Now, the danger in walking the neighborhood is that there's always a chance that you might encounter a neighbor.

And, it's not exactly an ideal circumstance to carry on a conversation when you're so worn out trying to keep up with Speedy Gonzales that you're practically slobbering down the front of your shirt and barely able to string a sentence together.

It was just a matter of time before the inevitable happened and we came across a neighbor, an athletic-looking lady who lived up the street.

The wife said something like, "Hey, how are you? Good to see you."

I intended to say something like, "Good to see you too." But I was totally out of breath and it came out sounding like, "Uuurgburgafayoo."

The neighbor just kind of stopped and looked at me, then went on with her conversation with the Mrs.

So, it took some time to get into a routine and build up some endurance, but eventually the walking was feeling more and more natural and we avoided any additional embarrassing episodes.

I was still pondering the future of my exercise when, virtually out of the blue, I dropped the bombshell on my wife that I wanted to start playing tennis with her.

She gave me a look that indicated that she found that idea about as appealing as having her toenails pulled out with pliers.

Even I'm not exactly sure where the idea came from. I mean, I had played some tennis earlier in my life, but probably hadn't picked up a racket in twenty years.

Finally, my wife reluctantly agreed to help me get started. And, in fairness, I completely understood her hesitancy.

You see, she has a fairly well-established circle of tennis friends built up over the years. Nice, classy people. Tennis tends to be a very social sport. I don't think I'm speaking out of turn here when I say that, especially for women, how you look and the way you act is almost as important as how you play.

And my behavior in public can be a little…shall we say, erratic, at times?

I mean, I don't suddenly peel off my clothes and run around naked or anything, but the occasional inappropriate humor or lame attempt at a practical joke is not unusual.

So, I think my wife saw a better-than-average chance of public embarrassment coming out of this whole endeavor.

Her fears quickly became a bit of a reality when, as part of my initial tennis training, she had me hitting with a ball machine.

The machine will continually feeds you balls, which will give you some good practice hitting ground strokes. Repetition is a big part of tennis, and the really good players have been participating from a young age and play regularly.

But after a while, hitting against a ball machine can get somewhat tedious, and tedium can sometimes bring out the worst in me.

So, after a little while, to spice things up a bit, I started adding sound effects when I hit the ball.

One was kind of like a martial arts "Kiai." (Think *Karate Kid*.)

Now, keep in mind that this practice session was on a public court with some of the wife's aforementioned classy friends nearby. So, the wife wasn't exactly wild about this new wrinkle.

Then I started addressing the ball.

Loudly.

So, each hit went something like this:

"COME TO PAPA" 'KIAI' [Hit]

"I'M ON TO YOU NOW" 'KIAI' [Hit]

"YOU'VE COME BACK FOR MORE, YOU FOOL" 'KIAI' [Hit]

After a few minutes of this, my wife had had enough, and she got up to leave, probably hoping people would think she didn't know who I was.

Of course, I saw an opportunity here as well.

"AHA, YOU'RE LEAVING, EH?" 'KIAI' [Hit]

"YOU FEAR MY DEVELOPMENT AS A PLAYER" 'KIAI' [Hit]

Later, I decided to challenge my skill and set the ball machine to send me overhead shots high in the air. On one such shot, I had to back up while looking up at the ball, and I tripped over my own feet.

So, there I was, flat on my back again, but the machine kept slinging balls over, and I kept on swinging and shouting.

"I'M NOT BEATEN YET" 'KIAI' [Miss]

"THINK I'VE GOT THIS ONE" 'KIAI' [Miss]

"OKAY, MAYBE NOT"

And so on. By this time, of course, the wife was long gone.

So, our early attempts at tennis together had, at best, mixed results.

In fairness to my wife, she mustered up enough courage to enter us into a mixed doubles league together. We did pretty well too, although it was just a recreational league and our competitive nature sometimes got the better of us. Some players in the league, who were just out for a nice leisurely tennis match, were a little scared by our intensity.

I personally think it's very important for dialysis patients to find a way to stay physically active.

It doesn't really matter what form your level of activity takes, but it is critical that it is something you enjoy. Human nature is such that we won't do something with consistency if we don't enjoy it.

You might start up a running routine, but I guarantee that if you think of running as torture, it won't last for long. You will inevitably start to think of reasons/excuses not to run one day. Then the next day, you'll think, hey, those excuses were pretty good yesterday, why not use them again today?

Before you know it, a month has gone by since you last ran.

Staying physically active is important for everyone, of course. But dialysis patients have the added challenge of days that are dominated by long treatments, and again, a lot of times we don't feel real well in between.

So, I've found it awfully easy to fall into a funk, where it feels like your life has two phases—dialysis and getting ready for dialysis.

Exercise and staying physically active is a great remedy. When I'm pushing myself in my workouts or playing in a tennis match, I'm not even thinking about dialysis.

I'll admit that it's a struggle to get motivated at times, but I feel much better after exercising. I also feel that my "mental well-being" has improved greatly.

And, of course, the long-term physical benefits of exercise are well-documented. For dialysis patients, helping to control your blood pressure is prime example.

In addition, a good sweat can help with the amount of fluid you need removed during your next treatment. Just don't compensate by guzzling too much Gatorade afterward.

Social Life

I think I hear laughing in the background.

No, I'm probably imagining it.

Wait, there it is again. Getting louder now.

Then, I realize, it's my wife.

"You're writing about social life??" she says, now close to hysterics.

"That's kind of like Rush Limbaugh writing about building relationships with women. Ha Ha Ha Ha."

"Very funny," I say.

"That's like Bernie Madoff writing about sound financial investing. Ha Ha Ha Ha."

"I'm writing about the effects dialysis can have on your social life, smart aleck."

That comment nearly sends her into convulsions.

When she can breathe again, she says, "You've got to be kidding. Like we had a social life *before* you went on dialysis. Ha Ha Ha Ha."

"C'mon now. It wasn't that bad."

"You're idea of a big night was a six-pack and *Championship Wrestling* on TV. Ha Ha Ha Ha."

"Hey, we went out sometimes."

More laughter.

"News flash! Running to Blockbuster to pick up the latest Claude Van Damme video does not constitute *going out*. Ha Ha Ha Ha."

Then she says, "What are you going to cover next, *Fixing Things around the House, Self-Taught*? Ha Ha Ha Ha."

Now I'm really offended.

I say, "I can hold my own around the house..."

She practically doubles over.

"Remember the time you almost electrocuted yourself trying to fix the intercom? Ha Ha Ha Ha. Or when you almost fell to your death changing the spotlight in our cathedral ceiling? Ooh, it's starting to hurt. Or, when you tried to fix the CD player and we ended up selling the pieces for scrap. Ha Ha Ha. Or when you..."

"Okay, okay. I get the point."

She can see that she's really hit a nerve here.

"Sorry honey. You go right back to writing about social life," she says, trying to control another outburst.

"After that," she continues, trying to look serious, "maybe you can write about something you really know a lot about."

I'm just waiting.

"Like maybe *Table Etiquette While Watching Sports on TV.* Ha Ha Ha Ha." The laughter starts all over again. "You can have a chapter on how to miss the TV when you throw your dessert across the room."

Then she says, "Be sure to share your thinking on how you're sure the players can hear you when you're yelling at the TV. Ha Ha Ha Ha."

Don't worry, she stopped laughing at the whole idea a couple of days later.

Okay, I'll be up front about it. Maybe having a social life is not exactly my forte.

And I admit that when it comes to romance, I'm something of a pinhead.

My wife and I could be in a setting with romantic potential, say a nice restaurant, and all I'm concerned with is getting a seat where I can see the TV and whether the special of the day includes onion rings.

My wife would be looking at me, as if to say, "Hey, knucklehead, remember me?"

And even then I don't get it.

I will misinterpret her look, and say something really classy like, "What's wrong honey? Your appetizer go bad?"

So, I think she lost hope of me getting it turned around romantically a while ago.

Then, toss in the time constraints of being on dialysis, and you really don't get a pretty picture.

Probably the biggest challenge of maintaining (or beginning) a social life while on dialysis is breaking out of the ruts we find ourselves falling into.

Our lives are sometimes so wrapped around our treatments that we tend to neglect other aspects of living.

Even on non-dialysis days, it's pretty hard to think of getting out and about when you are nauseated and totally exhausted.

So, it might take extra initiative to force yourself to be more active socially.

To my wife's point, we were always homebodies, even before dialysis wreaked havoc on our schedules.

Once though, literally out of the blue, we decided to have a "date weekend."

When we thought about it, it seemed like we hadn't been on a date since the Eisenhower Administration.

At the time, I was working about sixty hours a week and hmmm, let's see, what else was taking up a lot of the time in my life?

Oh yeah, I was on dialysis. That's it.

Anyone who's been on dialysis on the evening shift knows what it's like when you get home after treatment.

Your idea of a successful personal interaction is standing up and heading for bed without passing out.

Not exactly the height of romance.

So, we decided to go out to dinner on Friday, and since she's not a real movie fan (and I am), we compromised and decided to watch a movie at home.

(The compromise consisted of a pretty significant trade-off on my part. More on that later.)

We decided to go to a baseball game on Saturday.

And then we were scheduled to play mixed doubles in a round-robin tennis tournament on Sunday.

How's *that* for togetherness?

The two keys to arranging this weekend of fun were thinking out of the box and being able to negotiate what we wanted to do.

The negotiation part resulted in the trade-off that I mentioned earlier.

You see, my wife and I don't like the same kinds of movies, and she doesn't really like baseball, which I love.

So, I let her choose the movie for Friday night, and we agreed to go to the game the next day.

Now, it may sound like everything worked out just hunky-dory, but, as you might imagine, there's always a downside for someone in a negotiation.

The downside for me was that I had to sit through *Mama Mia*.

That was the movie she chose in exchange for going to the game.

I had a strong feeling that this was not a movie I would enjoy, but as soon as that kid started singing in the opening scene, I was like, oh boy, what have I done now?

About midway through the movie, which she really seemed to be enjoying, I was hoping I could fall asleep.

About three-quarters of the way through the movie, I was praying for sweet, blissful death.

Anyway, I got through the end of the movie without actually nosediving out the second story window of our house, which was looking like a pretty good alternative along the way.

But from that point on, after seeing that movie, whenever I hear a song from Abba I just about curl up into a fetal position.

As for the other nights in our date weekend, I found it interesting that my wife had to go through her series of warnings on my behavior before she would agree to be seen with me in public.

For the baseball game:

"No swearing, temper tantrums, or stamping your feet. And no threatening the life of the umpires or opposing manager."

For tennis:

"No throwing your racket, keep the cussing to a minimum, and no trying to tear down the net. AND STOP YELLING AT THE BALLS."

I'm happy to say that, given my set of instructions, we had ourselves a pretty good date weekend.

I may not be the best one to talk about issues with your social life while on dialysis, but I know you can actually have one, because I've seen *other* patients do it.

In one of my former dialysis centers, there was a very young person sitting next to me for treatment.

She was in her twenties and had apparently inherited kidney disease. You see instances of that every once in a while, and it really breaks your heart.

It's one thing for someone in the middle-age bracket to have to go through the rigors of dialysis. It's another for someone who's born with it or acquires it at a young age.

But this youngster wasn't going to let dialysis keep her down. Far from it.

When she was done with her sessions on the evening shift, she used to bound up out of her chair and practically run over to the scale to get her post-treatment weight.

One time, I asked her what was her rush.

She told me that she and her boyfriend were going out on the town and that she didn't want to be late.

I was like, "Going out on the town *after* dialysis?"

She said, "Yeah, c'mon Bob. It's only nine o'clock. The night is still young."

I said, "Oh yeah, right. Good point. Maybe I'll do something tonight too."

As if.

After she left and my treatment was over, I stumbled over to the scale, walking like Slim Pickens with a hernia—quite a contrast to her high-energy exit.

My legs were cramping, I had zero strength, and the potential of doing anything social was about the same as Charles Manson getting elected president.

I managed to drive myself home and my wife half carried me to our room where I promptly collapsed on my bed and didn't move until the next day.

My wife came in to look at me and said I looked so bad that she was about ready to order an autopsy.

Before I lost consciousness that night, I thought about the dialysis youngster out boogying the night away.

She was an inspiration to me in a way. I thought, it *is* possible to have a social life on dialysis.

Not easy…but possible.

Fitting some kind of social activity into a dialysis patient's calendar is similar to getting involved in some physical activity to stay active.

It can be very helpful in breaking up the monotony of living from treatment to treatment.

Being active socially is also like working out in that it takes some extra effort to do it. There are a lot of times that a patient just doesn't feel up to doing anything more active than flipping to another channel.

Making the effort to be social (and trust me, I know what kind of effort we're talking about here) can benefit a dialysis patient greatly. Falling into a rut is very easy when you're on dialysis.

Restlessness/Grumpiness

Those of you who require scientific proof before buying into a concept might not want to read this next section.

There's no science, no studies, and no evidence associated with this next theory.

Just a finely conceived notion that I am convinced is true.

Is that good enough for you?

Okay, here it is, and you might want to be sitting down.

I believe that people get grumpier as they get older.

Ground breaking thought, huh?

And, although the scientific proof may be lacking, I am not without evidence.

My evidence is that it's happening to me.

Right now.

Issues that used to breeze on by me without causing a stir now send me into orbit.

Even more of a concern, sometimes I'm grumpy for no apparent reason at all, giving more credence to the thought that it's just the onset of "Grumpy Old Man Syndrome."

So, you're probably wondering, what's this half-baked theory doing in this book?

Well, I'm also of the equally unscientific opinion that dialysis might be "greasing the skids" of this unfortunate trend.

I'll get to that later. First, the age thing.

Not only have I totally bought into this connection between age and grumpiness, but I think I understand *why* it happens.

(Again, the sitting position would be preferable here.)

Humans are creatures of habit. With few exceptions, we like to live a certain way.

As we age, it says here that most people get even more set in their ways, and it ticks us off when anything or anyone disrupts our way of life, even in a fairly insignificant way.

I've seen evidence of this grouchiness-aging connection in others as well.

A few years back, my wife and I were taking annual trips to Florida for vacation.

Now, don't get me wrong, I love Florida, but the average age there is just north of my area code.

And, if you would like to see some examples of grumpy old men and women, the Sunshine State is a treasure trove.

I remember one time I was working out in the gym located within the complex where we were staying.

The gym was really nothing fancy, just a converted room painted a gaudy shade of bright red that could just about bring on a seizure.

I was getting off an exercise bike when an older lady was coming my way in her workout clothes. She was one of those people who you couldn't determine her age just by looking at her.

Somewhere between seventy-five and 150.

Anyway, she came barreling toward the bike, and she brushed/shoved her way past me with her hand on my chest.

"Out of my way, sonny," she said.

I've always been taught to respect my elders, so I just said, "Yes ma'am."

A little later, she went over to the free weights, actually just fairly light dumbbells. I asked if she needed any help.

"I haven't needed any help since my husband died," she retorted sharply.

At that point, and old Abbott and Costello routine came to mind where Costello says, "Lady, he ain't dead, he's hiding."

I managed to keep that thought to myself and just went back to my workout.

Later, I could see that she was actually a very nice lady. We had bits and pieces of a normal conversation. It wasn't her fault that this grumpiness attack came on occasionally.

At one point in our discussion, she mentioned that she was a vegetarian.

I couldn't help myself.

I said, "You know what I could never figure out? If we're not supposed to eat animals, how come they're made out of meat?"

She just looked at me like she couldn't quite process that one.

Then, just as I was feeling better about my new friend, her grumpy personality came roaring back.

She looked up at the clock and abruptly announced, "You have five minutes."

I said, "Excuse me?"

"You have FIVE minutes!"

"What happens in five minutes?"

She looked exasperated and explained, as if I really should already know.

"Aerobics class starts in *five minutes.*"

"Oh, sure. Just slipped my mind. Sorry."

I was just about finished with my workout anyway. So I saved the indignity of her taking me by the collar and tossing me out on the sidewalk by just leaving quietly.

But, I could see that her personality was caught between being a basically nice person and getting annoyed at some interloper disrupting her well-established routine.

So, how does dialysis play into this dynamic?

Well, it's hard to describe, but dialysis brings on a sense of restlessness and, yes, irritability that could, and probably does, add to our grumpiness quotient.

It's a strange thing, and yet another conflict associated with the treatment. On the one hand, you often feel so sick you can barely move. On the other, dialysis can make you feel jumpy, restless, and generally suitable for the nearest straight jacket.

Not sure if it's something about the treatment itself that causes these feelings or if they are brought on by having to sit still in one position for hours on end. There is definitely restlessness *during* the treatment, which is understandable.

I mean, it's not easy being sick, miserable, and immobile all at the same time.

But, even when we're between treatments, the feeling of restlessness is prevalent.

Sometimes, you feel torn between the urge to just sack out or run around the block or do something more involved like write an opera or something.

This feeling can lead to some odd behavior that makes the people around you really wonder about your sanity.

You can be laying on your bed practically catatonic one minute and up ready to go jogging the next.

> One time, I had had a particularly rough treatment on a Friday night and still didn't feel very well the next day.
>
> I stayed in bed later than usual on Saturday morning, and my wife was checking on me frequently to make sure I was still breathing.

She went out to do something else and was coming back into our room, and we ran into each other with me dressed in my gym clothes ready to go for a workout.

She was looking at me in total amazement, and said, "What the heck do you think you're doing?"

Now I was all hyper.

"Going for a quick workout, maybe a jog, do some weights. Then I thought I'd rearrange the garage, or maybe put a new addition on the house."

She just rolled her eyes and shook her head.

Again, it's pretty hard for a non-dialysis patient to relate.

So, combine the aging factor with this inherent feeling of restlessness/irritability brought on by dialysis and you end up with some grumpy dudes (and dudettes) in and around your local dialysis centers.

It's best to give them plenty of space if you encounter them on an off day.

Feeling Old?

Since we've firmly concluded <wink wink> that dialysis adds to natural grumpiness as you get older, here's my next completely unscientific theory.

Dialysis makes you feel older than you are.

I guess you can just about pencil my name in on that Nobel Prize now.

Well, okay, maybe not.

But, when you're on dialysis, you definitely have to fight off a sense that life is passing you by. Your treatments are long and frequent, a total of four to four-and-a-half hours, three times a week.

You build your schedule and your life around your treatments.

This grueling schedule seems to make time go by extremely fast.

Say your treatments are scheduled in the morning. You go in first thing, wipe out your entire morning, and feel weak and sick the rest of that day.

You start feeling better the next day, re-hydrate carefully, and by the following evening you're fit and ready to move forward.

Except then, it's time for your next treatment the next morning, and the cycle starts all over again.

Then, before you know it, the week is gone.

Seems like you start on dialysis, you blink your eyes, and suddenly, you've been on it for five years.

Now, I know that, for most people, life seems to go by faster as you age anyway. But I really think the regimentation required for dialysis treatments adds to and magnifies this feeling.

Plus, let's face it, these treatments make us feel like our get-up-and-go has got-up-and-went. They can really sap your strength.

I was on dialysis while working my last couple of years in my corporate job. Perhaps some of my feelings about accelerated aging were also impacted by the fact that most of the people I worked with my last few years were much younger than me.

One time, I was participating in a United Way event at the office. Some of the other senior people and I were serving pancakes in exchange for donations to the United Way.

I came across a younger associate who I hadn't seen in a while, and I just casually said, "So, how's it going?"

Big mistake.

I'm paraphrasing here, but her response was something like:

"Oh the other night, I was on my Facebook, and my boyfriend tweeted me, so I had to text him back, and he was like, LOL LOL, and he wanted me to catch this tricked-up video on YouTube, so I sent him a new string, and then…"

I was getting a little dizzy, so I interrupted.

"Well, that's great, but the line is building up behind you here."

She said, "No worries, I'll catch up with you later."

I thought, it would be more like me catching up to you since you left me so far in the dust back there.

After I got 'off duty,' I was chatting with some people when I saw the same girl making a beeline for me. I had the horrible thought that she wanted to continue that earlier conversation.

So, I ditched my coffee and said, "Sorry, gotta go," mid-conversation and I high-tailed it out of there.

Also, most mornings when I went to work, I made it a point to climb the stairs instead of take the elevator. My office was on the third floor of a three-story building.

I was going up the stairs at what I considered to be a pretty good pace, but one time, some employee who looked like he was about twelve went buzzing by me at about double my speed and made it look effortless.

And, to add insult to injury, as he sped past me he said, "Oh, excuse me, sir."

The next day, as I was climbing the stairs again, I heard someone coming up fast behind me.

I glanced back and realized it was the same kid.

I had to fight off the urge to stick my foot out and send the kid hurling over the rail.

Yes, I think working around younger people definitely added to my feeling of being old before my time.

I experienced a similar situation when I would go to the gym.

Usually, I'm by far the oldest person in the gym, especially when I go in the morning.

I'd run away with the "Most Likely to Keel Over" vote among my peers.

And, now I have to fight off my testosterone-fueled competitive urges.

It used to be that I wouldn't allow anyone to run faster or lift more weight than me; I had to be right up there with them.

Now, with my dialysis-sapped strength, I'm lucky to get through a minimal routine without requiring hospitalization.

There are some generalizations in this section that border on criminal and may not apply to all dialysis patients.

I can only speak to how the rigors of dialysis have affected me and how I have dealt with these difficult treatments over the past several years.

I certainly felt the onset of the "Grumpy Old Man" syndrome *before* I went on dialysis. This feeling came on somewhere in my early fifties. Suddenly, you would have to peal me off the walls over things that I found trivial before.

But since starting dialysis, my personal opinion is that having to go through these treatments and feeling lousy all the time has made matters worse. For me, the feelings of restlessness, grouchiness, and accelerated aging, if not *caused* by dialysis, have at least been *magnified* by it.

I'm not trying to blame the treatments for an inherent personality flaw—as convenient as that would be. I know that some of this distemper is just part of who I am. If I had to put a percentage on reasons for getting grumpier, it'd be like sixty percent just naturally grumpy old me and forty percent dialysis.

And heaven knows, I started feeling the effects of aging long before dialysis entered the picture.

In my younger years, I was a very fast runner. But starting about when I turned forty, you could clock me with a sundial.

I used to think of myself as having above-average agility, but by the time I retired, it was all I could do to keep from being run over by the mail cart in the office.

I admit that my opinions about grumpiness and aging are generalizations. There may well be some perfectly well-adjusted dialysis patients who walk around in a perpetual happy mood all the time.

I haven't met any, but I acknowledge the possibility that they're out there.

My theory does *not* mean that if you know a happy, peppy person and they discovered they needed dialysis, they would turn into an insufferable curmudgeon the day after they started treatment.

The following week, maybe.

No, just kidding.

But the treatment can do a number on you physically over time. If you're a dialysis patient and you find yourself getting a little grouchier or start feeling like you're aging before your time, don't worry too much.

It's just a natural part of the process.

Working

Disability Bound?

I'll never forget one of my initial conversations with a doctor when I first started dialysis. I was still in the hospital at the time.

The doctor was giving me the lowdown on what my life was going to be like from now on. (Little did I know at the time that he really didn't have a clue.)

"I don't see how you can continue to work," he said.

My brilliant comeback was, "Huh?"

"People on dialysis usually don't work."

"Why not?"

"Well, because they can't. They feel sick all the time; there are complications from the treatments. And, dialysis doesn't fit well with a work schedule."

Keep in mind that I was in my early thirties, and I was extremely career-minded. I had gone to college; in fact, I had an advanced degree. And I had a corporate job with a big company.

So, to put it mildly, I was not exactly a receptive audience for his message.

"Well, in that case," I continued, "think they need any help clearing the breakfast dishes downstairs?"

"How's that again?" said the doctor.

"You know. Washing dishes. Isn't that a good fallback for people who can't work?"

"I don't think you understand."

"No, I don't think YOU understand."

I was getting a little hot under the collar at this point. So, I went on with my rant.

"If I thought I was going to blow tens of thousands of dollars on my education without working, I would have at least gone to the track instead and had some fun with the money."

"No wait…"

"No, YOU wait! You mean to tell me that the last several years I've spent in corporate America trying to work my way up the ladder, I could have been on the beach instead?"

"Ummm, well…"

"What a bummer. I might be an Olympic-level surfer by now. And think of all the bikinis I've missed out on seeing."

He just sat back and rolled his eyes.

"Are you finished?" he asked.

"Not quite. I've got another question for you."

He just raised his eyebrows warily in response.

"Do you think the people downstairs use the kind of dish-washer soap that doesn't dry out your hands?"

At this point, the doctor had had enough fun and pretty much gave up on the conversation.

"I'll come back another time," he said.

"You'd better call first. I might be on the early shift downstairs."

Then, he just nodded his head in resignation and left.

As soon as he was out the door, I promptly proceeded to start freaking out.

I began wondering…was he right?

I had just had my first couple of experiences with the dialysis treatment, and yes, they took up an awful lot of time. And yes, I'd already experienced some of the side effects.

My second treatment in my blood pressure dropped. One second I was having a conversation with the dialysis technician and the next I had fuzzed out, and the technician had pushed the head of my chair all the way back so I was practically upside down.

My first thought when I came to was did I die and come back as a vampire bat?

Then, I was looking upside down at the technician and a nurse.

"You passed out; we're giving you some saline," said the nurse.

Providing saline and putting you in a position so that blood runs to your head are the first things they do to someone who zonks out during a treatment.

Another time early on, I got my introduction to cramping.

Nobody had warned me that I might cramp during treatment, so this experience really took me by surprise.

I didn't have the fistula vessel in my arm yet, so they were using that wonderful gangly-looking catheter in my upper chest for my treatment.

One of the good things about the catheter—and trust me, there aren't many—is that it allows you to have both hands free. Once they start using the fistula, you have to keep the arm with the vessel as still as possible.

I was taking advantage of being able to use both my hands by doing a crossword puzzle. I've found that puzzles make the time of my treatment go by really fast.

So, I'm in my hospital bed, dialyzing and doing my puzzle when suddenly the pencil flew out of my hand and landed clear across the room.

What the heck was that? I wondered.

I was going to reach over and signal for the nurse to get my pencil—still pretty much unaware of what was happening.

When I reached for the button, my other hand seized, and I hit the button to lower the foot of my bed instead.

So, I was sliding down toward the bottom of my bed, and when I tried to use my feet to stop my slide, I lost control of both legs as well.

Fortunately for me, the nurse came in at that point. She just stopped in the doorway, shocked at what she saw.

I was crumpled up in a ball at the foot of the bed, trying to squirm my way back up.

I probably looked like an inchworm with an elevated blood alcohol level.

She was like, "What's going on?" as she came over to fix the bed.

Even my mouth wasn't working right.

"The button hit the pencil wrong, and I almost fell on the nurse," I said.

She just looked at me.

It seemed like a delayed reaction, but then the pain of the cramps finally registered, and I said something like, "HOOOH OOOOO EEEE YAAA!!"

"Are you cramping?" she asked.

"YAAAAA. CRAMPING. EEEEYAAAA!!"

She gave me some saline and pushed on my feet and hands as best she could until the cramps cleared up.

Now, back to the freaking out discussion over my job.

I really wondered at that point if I would be able to work. I mean, what if something like that cramping episode happened in the middle of a meeting, which was a very real possibility as I would find out in the future.

Then I thought, what am I thinking? *Of course* I'm going back to work. I'll find a way to cope.

That thought about returning was a lot more confident than I really felt; I was actually very worried.

The next day, the social worker came in.

"I'm here to help you with your application for disability," she said.

"Disability?"

"Yes, you know, for when you leave the hospital."

She was a nice, older lady. So, I couldn't really follow my first impulse, which was to tell her where she could stick those application papers.

"No, I'm going back to work," I said.

She just looked at me as if I had told her there were aardvarks living in the ceiling.

"Work? Haven't you talked to Dr. [So and So]?"

"Yes, he was going to set me up with a dishwashing gig downstairs."

"What?"

"Never mind. Look, I made the decision that I'm going back to work, and that's all there is to it."

She said, "You know, they haven't even determined the length of your treatments yet. It could be four hours. Could be longer. How are you going to work with those treatments? And hasn't anyone told you about the side effects?"

"Told me? I've already been a vampire bat who won an Olympic gold in pencil throwing."

"Excuse me?"

"Never mind."

I then went on to explain that I was too young and had invested too much in my career to quit and go on disability.

As far as dealing with the schedule and the side effects, well, I really didn't know yet how I was going to handle those.

I was like the blockheaded guy who's lost while driving his wife around. When she asks if he knows where he's going, he says, "No, but we'll find out when we get there."

That's how I felt about the scheduling and side effect issues. I would find out how I was going to deal with them when the opportunity arose.

I encountered several more people during my hospital stay who tried to "explain" how it wasn't possible for me to work while I was on dialysis.

They were met with varying forms of sarcasm, sick humor, rudeness, and derision.

So, finally, I was close to getting discharged and that doctor came back—an act of courage on his part.

He sat down and tried to take a reasoned approach with me.

"So, I hear you're not exactly accepting of the limitations of life on dialysis," he said.

I said, "Look Doc, I accept that there are going to be limits, but I wasn't put on this earth to go on disability. If I can't do my current job, then I'll find one that I can do."

We then went on to have a pretty good conversation about potential issues, problems, and more importantly, solutions for to my new lifestyle.

I don't mean to make it sound like I'm the only one who decided to continue working after starting dialysis. That is far from the truth.

But a relatively small percentage of dialysis patients are able to continue to work. And I certainly understand why the majority of patients are unable to continue working.

There are many trials and tribulations associated with working while you're on dialysis. Some are easy to deal with, some… not so much.

Going Back To Work

The one piece of advice I can give about going back to work after starting dialysis is: Don't rush it.

In other words, don't do what I did.

I had additional conversations with that doctor who told me I wouldn't be able to work anymore. When it became clear to him that I was going to do it anyway, he started emphasizing the physical and mental toll that dialysis can take.

He had switched his focus to trying to talk me into taking it slow once I did go back.

Now, whether it was a sense of pride, my desire to get back to a somewhat normal lifestyle, or just plain stupidity, I pretty much disregarded everything he told me.

He said that after I was discharged from the hospital, I should plan on taking four to six weeks to get my strength back before returning to work.

So, what did I do? I went back after one week.

The doctor also said that once I did go back to work, I should start on half days and work my way back to full days.

Bzzzz. I started right back on a full-time schedule.

The doctor said he wanted to see me once a week for a while after I started working again.

So, what did I do? Blew off the first couple of appointments and moseyed back in to see him after about a month.

Not exactly a model patient.

But again, I emphasize—*don't do what I did.*

Before I got out of the hospital, the staff had to be sure that I had a place to go for my ongoing treatments in a dialysis center. I needed to have dialysis during the evening shift (or third shift) because I was going to be working during the day.

Unfortunately, the staff could only find me a seat in a center about twenty-five miles from my home for that particular shift. I wasn't exactly filled with joy about making that drive, especially *after* my treatments, but it worked with my work schedule, so I went with it.

After I got out of the hospital, I took a week off and was just about ready to shoot myself with boredom. So I thought about working and thought, well, how bad can it be? I'll go back to work next week and just take it easy.

Right.

So, I made my triumphant return to work the following week looking and feeling like something the cat dragged in.

Now, I should make a point here that will help clarify a few things about my work life.

I'm not one to talk a whole lot about my personal life, especially an illness, at work.

The people at work closest to me, like the people in my organization, all obviously knew what was going on with my kidney failure and hospital stay. But outside of that group, the rest of the company only knew that I had been out for a couple of weeks.

I wasn't the type who would walk into my first meeting back and just stand up and say,

"Hey guess what everybody? My kidneys conked out and I need three nasty dialysis treatments per week to stay alive! How about me, huh?"

No, I pretty much kept all my medical issues to myself and just tried to cope.

My first day back, I felt semi-okay early on, but things got progressively worse during the day.

You tend to forget that a hospital stay of any length really drains you. Plus, dialysis really drains you.

So, by the end of my first morning, I guess you could say that I was pretty drained.

Then I went down to my company's cafeteria for lunch. I was still learning about the renal diet, so I was a little gun shy about deciding what I wanted to eat.

I ended up with a plain turkey sandwich on white bread and a small cup of water—real exciting stuff.

Anyway, I sat down in the cafeteria with some people I knew. Everyone welcomed me back. Most of this group kind of knew what was happening with me.

Then I made a big mistake.

I said, "So, how do you think I look?"

Everyone shifted in their seats a little.

"Great!"

"Awesome!"

"Fit as a fiddle!"

"Like you were on the wrong end of a train derailment."

The last comment came from a guy, of course. And he was the only one really telling me the truth. Because, if I looked even close to the way I felt, then the picture wasn't pretty.

But I foolishly tried to stick it out for the rest of the afternoon.

By the end of that first day, I was practically gasping for breath and about ready to be carted off on a stretcher.

I remember thinking, well, maybe that doctor who tried to tell me that I wouldn't be able to work wasn't so dumb after all.

Maybe resting a little more or starting back part-time would have been better than practically having to crawl home after my first day back.

It took me a while to get back in the swing of things and even close to feeling like my old self again.

I was eventually able to build my strength up and adjust to my new schedule.

Before dialysis, I was always one of those hopeless people who got to work early and left late.

Now, my treatments were scheduled to start at 4:30 PM, and I had to account for that drive to the treatment center that was twenty-five miles away.

(Many of my treatments *actually started* at five in the evening or beyond because I was late, but that's a whole 'nother story.)

So, three days a week—Monday, Wednesday, and Friday—I had to leave work earlier than normal to get down to my dialysis center on time. That really took some adjusting on my part.

The people who I worked with who *didn't* know about my kidney failure were really wondering where the heck I was going when I left early. They still thought of me as someone who always worked late. And, again, my personality was such that I let them wonder. I wasn't going to clarify anything for them.

Besides, I always got to the office earlier in the morning than everybody else, so I could make up any lost time.

Because of my corporate position, I attended a lot of meetings. Fortunately for me, I was in a senior position by this point in my career, which meant that I could request that most late meetings on a treatment day be rescheduled.

Every once in a while, there was a late meeting that I couldn't get out of or reschedule, so occasionally I would either have my treatment that morning instead of the afternoon or go in for treatment the next day.

After I'd been back to work for a couple of weeks, I got the sense that I could, in fact, continue working full time. There were times when I felt really awful, and I faced many dialysis-related issues, but I also came to realize that working was great therapy for many of my ills.

I still felt that I could do my job, that I could still *outperform* by my expectations and by my company's standards and that I could make up any time lost to account for my dialysis treatment schedule.

Honestly, if I didn't feel that way, I would have considered resigning. I was determined that I wasn't going to cheat my company. I felt that as I continued to get stronger after my hospital stay, I was going to get back to my pre-dialysis levels of productivity and performance.

So, I deemed the early trial of going back to work a success.

Of course, there would be many more tribulations going forward.

Feeling Ill

Among the many issues that come and go as you try to go back to work after starting dialysis, there's one that really affects you *all* the time.

That is that, for the most part, you always feel like crap.

Hope I didn't bog you down in technical terms there.

Earlier, I described the vicious cycle that you go through when you're on in-center hemodialysis. Remember? Just when you start feeling better, it's time for another treatment?

Although the machine does a good job of cleaning your blood, it can't replace the twenty-four-hour operation of a normally functioning kidney. As such, you never really feel like you are one hundred percent, or back to how you felt when your kidneys were working.

So, it was definitely an adjustment for me to be at work feeling poorly basically all the time.

My job required a high degree of energy, and sometimes I really had to work hard to muster it up.

In addition, remember we're talking about Mr. Clandestine Dialysis Patient here.

I wasn't about to let on to anyone at work that I wasn't feeling well.

I went to meetings, held conference calls, had one-on-ones with associates in my organization, and worked at my desk—all the while fighting off the urge to just upchuck and get it over with.

But, I think of myself as a pretty tough critic of my own performance, and when I thought about it, I didn't feel like my work performance had suffered.

Perhaps even more importantly, I didn't get the vibe or, for that matter, direct feedback that anyone else thought so either.

That's not to say that my work situation was perfect and without pitfalls.

There were times when that dialysis-related, old-age, don't-feel-well grumpiness reared its ugly head.

I had an exchange with a young member of my organization that made me think I should be locked away to prevent further human contact.

The employee came into my office to drop off a routine report—a frequent occurrence during a normal day.

I was reviewing a contract at the time, but when I saw her out of the corner of my eye, I barked, "WHAT IS THAT?"

She nearly jumped out of her skin.

She looked at me wide-eyed, and said meekly,

"It's the Monthly Category Profitability Report."

"WHY ARE YOU BRINGING THAT IN HERE NOW?"

She backed up a few steps and said, "It's due today at noon."

"SO WHAT? WHAT TIME IS IT?"

"Umm, 11:45."

At this point, I could tell by the look on her face that she was thinking that my numbers weren't quite adding up, if you know what I mean.

That brought me back to my senses, and I calmed down some.

She was still inching back toward the door, as if she expected me to tear off my clothes, let out a war cry, and take her as human sacrifice.

I was somewhat embarrassed by my little outburst.

"Okay, good job getting it in on time," I said.

She said, "Sure thing," and then high-tailed it out of there like she was being chased by a guy with an axe.

Afterward, I was thinking, okay, what was that all about?

Who was that crazy person pretending to be me just now?

Later, I went to her office, apologized for my outburst, and tried to be overly nice to her for the next few days.

She still looked a little wary when I talked to her, though. And I'm not sure she was buying the too-nice routine.

She was probably thinking, does this guy have multiple personalities or what?

What is this, *Sybill Part 2: The Winged-Out Corporate Executive*?

So as much as I had to adjust to my new working life on dialysis, to a certain extent, others had to make adjustments as well.

The morning after a tough treatment could be particularly challenging. A bout of cramping, or bleeding, or nausea, or restlessness that keeps you awake all night can really make getting up and going to work (early) an ordeal.

I'll admit, there were times when I wondered if I could continue to work full time.

But, just as I was wondering if I was ready to nosedive into the junk heap, I had a true inspiration in the form of another person.

Around that time, I had a discussion with another dialysis patient that led to my looking at a guy at work as an inspiration.

In my discussion with this other patient, I contended that as bad as dialysis patients have it, there are *many* people who are much worse off. The other patient thought that being on dialysis was akin to being treated for cancer.

I was like, sorry bro. Not even close.

I knew a young guy working in my office who was, in fact, being treated for cancer. He didn't work in my organization, and I didn't really know him that well, but he was friends with some people who worked for me, so they kept me informed about his situation.

He was in his thirties with a wife and two young kids.

The guy kept trying to work through the cancer treatment process, and when people described what he was going through, I was amazed.

The cancer had spread to his brain, and he had lost feeling on the right side of his face.

He kept coming to work.

His doctors told him that he would go blind within a month and that he had a fifty percent chance of living through the year.

He kept coming to work.

In fact, he kept coming to work for as long as it was physically possible, and, from what I understand, his work performance hardly suffered at all.

I told my dialysis peer about this remarkable young man. Then I said, "Think if this cancer patient had the option of three treatments a week to cure all his major symptoms that he wouldn't jump at the chance? You bet he would," I said.

I realized that as tough as we dialysis patients have it, there are, in fact, many people who are *much* worse off.

And, I couldn't help admiring that young man, with everything that he was going through to fight his cancer, continuing to work and doing a good job.

He eventually lost his fight with cancer, but he remained an inspiration to me until the day that I retired.

That's why I managed to get up early every morning, even after a tough treatment or a sleepless night, and haul my sorry butt to work.

Because I could.

So, after adjusting to my work schedule, I decided to take a new tack mentally in dealing with my dialysis-related issues.

I was going to *ignore* how bad I felt.

Easier said than done? Yes, perhaps.

But taking a positive attitude kept me from getting hung up about how lousy I felt.

I applied additional focus and concentration on my work, which served the dual purpose of helping me forget about how I felt and increasing my personal productivity.

In business you are ultimately evaluated by your productivity. By all measures, my department and I were highly productive my last few years.

And, by the way, those years went by fast.

Work Issues

Hopefully, I've given you a flavor of what life on dialysis is like. The way you feel is largely hit or miss—some days are just better than others.

Just like work, dialysis is a long-term prospect. The two need to coexist, so you have to build a workable pattern, incorporating both into your day-to-day routine.

Of course, if you have the kind of job, as I did, that is anything but routine, it can be challenging at times to work around your set dialysis schedule.

And, the other physical complications of dialysis can cause a variety of issues that can disrupt your hopes for a normal working life.

Managing work and dialysis, there were some days when it just seemed like everything was going wrong.

One day, I had been through a tough treatment the night before. My vessel had infiltrated, causing my arm to swell to twice its normal size. I had experienced dizziness, nausea, itching, and cramping. I had that post-dialysis restlessness that kept me up most of the night.

In other words, when I dragged myself out of my bed the next morning, it was not a pretty picture.

Even after showering, shaving, and getting dressed, I felt completely disheveled and couldn't shake the feeling that I was forgetting something or that something was amiss before I left for work.

But, somehow I managed to get myself to the office, no doubt looking like death warmed over.

I figured having some coffee might help, so I went down to the coffee shop and got myself a cup.

When I got up to the register, I reached in my pocket, and thought, oh no.

I had forgotten to bring my money.

I normally keep my cash in a money clip and put it in my pocket in the morning. But in my post bad-treatment daze, I had left it on my bureau that day.

So, I greeted the cashier, who I knew pretty well, and I pulled out my debit card.

She was just looking at me.

"You're paying eighty-nine cents for a cup of coffee with a debit card?" she asked.

I tried to make it look like there was some strategic thinking involved.

"Well, yeah, you know, trying to consolidate all my purchases and take advantage of the buying consolidation."

Pretty weak.

So, I slinked off to go back to my office.

I didn't feel up to taking the stairs, so I walked over to the elevator, pushed the down button instead of up, and had to go up to the third floor via the basement.

When I got back to my office, I thought, okay, well at least I'll be able to cherish my morning coffee.

As I took the lid off and brought the cup up to my lips, I forgot about the swelling in my arm and spilled the coffee down the front of my shirt.

Oh, the cuss words that came out. It would make my mama ashamed.

So, in addition to having a general feeling of being out of sorts, I now had a coffee stain roughly the shape of Brazil on my dress shirt.

A little later, that buddy of mine who's always brutally honest came waltzing into my office.

"You look awful," he said.

"Yeah, well, so do you," I replied cleverly. "I had a tough night last night."

"Really? Were you wearing that shirt at the time?"

"Huh?"

"That stain is starting to resemble South America."

"No, I spilled my coffee this morning."

"Uh huh. Are you wearing different shoes?"

"What?"

"Looks like one is black and one is brown."

I looked down.

"Oh crap, I have a meeting with [the Chief Financial Officer] this afternoon."

"I wouldn't recommend that. See if you can reschedule—unless you're making a pitch for the VP of Homeless Relations job."

Everybody's a comedian.

Fortunately, I had an extra dress shirt in my closet that I kept for just such emergencies.

So, I went to the men's room and changed my shirt.

Later that morning, my assistant came into my office, and we were just chitchatting.

Suddenly, she said, "Is that blood?"

"What?"

"Is that blood on your sleeve?"

I looked down.

"Uh oh," I said.

"Not only is your sleeve a mess, but, unless I'm seeing things, the spot is getting bigger," she said.

Turns out, one of my insertion sites had given way under the bandage, and I was bleeding all over the place.

So, I put pressure on the site to stop the flow. And of course I had extra bandages in my desk that I kept for just such...well you know.

She said, "Don't worry, you can just change into your spare shirt."

"This is my spare shirt."

"Uh oh."

So, she went out to her desk and dug in her purse and came up with some spot remover towelettes.

(I'm frequently amazed at how many different things are in women's purses, but that's another story.)

Surprisingly, these towelettes worked pretty well, and we got the blood stains off of my sleeve.

When I pulled my sleeve up, however, she nearly fainted at the sight of my arm.

"What the heck happened there?"

"Ah, I infiltrated last night."

"Oh boy."

She could sense that this was just going to be one of those days.

I still wasn't feeling that well when a little later another associate stopped by my office.

"Bob, can you come into the conference room for a minute? We need your take on something."

I said, "Oh sure." I stood up, got a wicked cramp in my leg, almost fell down, and started limping toward my door.

"Are you okay?" he said.

I didn't want to go into the real story, so I just made something up.

"Oh, yeah," I said as I staggered along. "Just tweaked a hammy playing tennis the other day."

He just looked at me, not quite sure he was buying it.

As I limped past my assistant's desk, she just looked down and shook her head.

Anyway, I managed to get through the morning without any further disasters and reached lunchtime.

I felt like I should minimize the time I was seen in public, so I asked my assistant to just bring something back to my office.

Of course, consistent with the day's proceedings, the cafeteria didn't have my usual fare, so my assistant had to improvise and get something else.

"I hope you can have this. I know the list of things you can eat is shorter than Herve Villechaize after a crewcut," she said.

"Yeah, it'll be fine."

It just so had it that, that day I was supposed to start taking a new prescription for phosphorous, and the pill was supposed to be taken with meals.

So, I popped a pill with lunch, but what I wasn't told was that these little beauties can make you nauseous as a side effect. And I was already nauseous.

Later that afternoon, I was in my meeting with the CFO, and about mid-sentence, the nausea kicked into gear.

It was something like, "And these charts show [urp]…"

"Are you okay?" asked the CFO.

I was thinking, boy a lot of people have asked me that today.

Of course, I tried to mask my discomfort.

"Oh yeah, no big deal. So as I was saying [urrumpurmuff]…"

"What was that?"

"Oh nothing. Hey, how about we take a quick break? I think you're really gonna be impressed later…" I said with a big forced smile.

So, we took a break, and, with my mismatched shoes, I bolted for the men's room.

I did make it through the rest of the meeting. Afterward, feeling tired and beaten down, I managed to practically crawl back to my office.

My assistant was getting ready to leave for the day.

She came in and looked at me sympathetically.

"Are you okay?"

I just sat there thinking, here we go again.

"You look like you could use about three days of sleep," she said. "Your complexion's a little on the green side. Kind of like Herman Munster."

I gave the stock answer, "Yeah, I'm fine. Just a little tired."

She just rolled her eyes. "Right. A little tired. Like saying Elvis was a little chubby."

My assistant was great. She provided great support and was a friend as well. But I could never put anything by her.

"Okay, I've felt like crap all day, and just about everything has gone wrong today," I said.

"Why don't you just cut your losses and go home before you burn the building down or something."

"Nah, just going to stick it out a while longer. Besides," I continued with a lot more cheer than I really felt, "what else could go wrong today?"

She just looked at me doubtfully and left.

Later, as I was getting ready to leave, I thought I'd take the stairs going down, since I'd skipped them coming in that morning.

As I was walking down, I started feeling pain in my knee joints.

I thought, oh no.

I had experienced previous bouts with gout that had caused serious joint pain, and I was afraid it was coming on again.

But I was already halfway down the stairs, and it was too late to turn back.

So, I continued hobbling down, with the occasional yelp of pain, and holding onto the rail for dear life.

Someone, who I didn't know, stopped beside me.

"Are you okay?"

I thought, geez, now complete strangers are asking me.

I didn't know why, but I had to come up with a different story from the earlier one.

"Uh, yeah. Just an old football injury acting up heh heh."

She just looked at me as if to say, "Yeah, we'll go with that," and moved on.

As I was limping out to my car, I was thinking, watch, now the car won't start. Or, someone stole my tires or something.

But the car was in one piece, started up fine, and I got myself home without further incident.

"How was your day?" asked the wife.

I just kind of laughed in response.

Days like that didn't happen that often, but when they did, they made me wonder anew about continuing to work while I was on the Big D.

Another potential pitfall at work was my blood pressure running low on days after treatments, which could cause dizziness at unfortunate times.

This became more of an issue as I made it up through the ranks and had more opportunities for public speaking or presenting to large groups.

One such time, it was a "day after," and I was scheduled to speak to a group of about 600 people.

The room was set up auditorium style and before speaking, I was sitting in the front row. The current speaker was introducing me, saying nice things.

I was getting all psyched up. When the speaker finished with the introduction, I stood up to go to the podium.

Too fast. Got dizzy. Came close to cratering. Almost did a face-plant on the stage.

In a way, I was fortunate by not fainting outright. I had become almost accustomed to dealing with dizzy spells from other low blood pressure episodes after treatments. I knew not to panic when I walked up to the stage and that the dizziness would probably pass.

So, I kept calm, caught my breath, and was able to complete the presentation without falling down.

As I was up on the stage, I was thinking about a previous incident at home where I did actually pass out and thought, phew, dodged a bullet this time.

The original episode happened on a night after I got home from a treatment. I didn't have too much fluid taken off, but my BP was borderline low when I left the center.

I had dinner and was just chilling out watching TV with the wife.

After eating, the digestion process can draw blood towards the stomach, which can lower your blood pressure even further and also lessen the amount of blood going to your head.

Of course, I wasn't cognizant of that at the time, and as I stood up to go to the kitchen, the next thing I knew, I was like, "Dude, how'd the room get sideways?"

Then I realized, I was lying on my side on the kitchen floor with my wife standing above me, shaking me by the shoulders trying to bring me out of it.

Turns out, I had stood up too fast, and the combination of the dialysis-lowered BP along with the digestion of my dinner caused me to black out.

My wife remembered looking my way as I was heading to the kitchen, then looking back and wondering where I went.

Splayed out on the floor was probably not high on her list of possibilities, but there I was.

So, this all went through my mind in the aftermath of my dizzy spell heading up to the stage.

Being nauseous in the CFO's office was hardly the only time that happened either.

There were many times that I had to step out of a meeting to keep from a mid-meeting hurl.

That has a tendency to really disrupt a meeting agenda.

On occasion, I had to participate in a business meeting via conference call while I was actually on dialysis. If, for whatever reason, a meeting couldn't be rescheduled and I needed to be a part of it, my choices were to have my treatment another time—not always possible and usually not recommended—or participate in a conference call while being treated.

Now, calling in wasn't preferable for me. I've always found that personally attending a meeting is best, but sometimes participating via phone just couldn't be avoided.

Of course, participating in a meeting while you're on dialysis presents some pretty unique situations. You have to hope and pray that nothing goes wrong during the treatment.

During one such dialysis treatment, I dialed in to participate in a meeting via conference call while I was actually
hooked up to the machine.

BEEP-BEEP-BEEP-BEEP

Suddenly, my machine alarm went off.

"What was that?" someone on the conference call
asked.

Once again, my improvisational skills were put to the
test.

"Oh, a garbage truck nearby just went down the street
backward. Imagine that!" I said.

Okay, maybe improv is not my thing.

The reason for the alarm was that my veinous pressure
dropped below its minimum threshold. This meant that
the blood returning to my body wasn't going in as fast as
it should have been, which sets off a really annoying alarm
on the machine.

An attendant came over.

"Your veinous pressure is too low. We're going to have
to pull the tape and adjust your needles," she said.

Of course, someone on the call overheard.

"Uh...Bob? Who is pulling what tape? And did I hear that someone's adjusting your needles?"

Oh boy.

So, I managed to gloss over that, and, for a while, we got back to business on the call.

Then, just my luck, it had to be one of those treatments where everybody in the dialysis center and their brother had something they needed to discuss with me.

First, the head nurse.

"We want to be sure everyone is familiar with the emergency evacuation plan," she said.

Someone on the call: "Are you okay? Where are you being evacuated from?"

Clever me: "No big deal. My personal trainer was just saying where to go in case a tornado hit heh heh."

Then, the dietician.

"I wanted to talk to you about your hemoglobin," she said.

Someone on the call: "Did someone just say that they wanted to talk to you about a *hobgoblin?*"

Witty little me: "Oh yeah, we're getting a jump start on our plans for Halloween."

"But Bob, it's only June."

"Hey, don't you ever plan in advance? My wife buys all our Christmas wrap off the clearance displays in January heh heh…"

And, of course, the social worker from the center didn't want to get left out.

"I had a question about your insurance," she said.

Someone on the call: "Why is someone asking about your insurance? Were you in an accident?"

Frustrated, at-the-end-of-his-ability-to-improvise me: "Something like that. This whole call is turning into a train wreck."

And on it went.

There were many challenges to working dialysis into my normal business routine.

As I established my work routine, I felt like I had to put in extra effort to make up for the days when I would leave early for my treatment.

Don't get me wrong, my *total* work hours were probably in the top ten percent of associates at my level. I was usually leaving the office at 4:00 to 4:15 PM on dialysis days. On non-treatment days, I was at work until whenever.

But, as I mentioned earlier, I came into the office super early *every* day, even after a bad treatment, which, of course, meant that I had to get up early every day, even after getting home late the night before.

As a result, there were many mornings when I got to the office not exactly feeling fit and pink. And my challenge was to make these extra hours in the morning super productive.

I was in a decision-making position. But, I decided early on that, if I wasn't feeling one hundred percent, I would put off any major decisions until I was feeling better.

What led me to that conclusion was an occurrence soon after I started the Big D. I was in at my usual time on a Tuesday morning after a particularly brutal treatment on Monday night.

Let's see…what did I have happen during that treatment? There was…oh never mind. You know all the bad things that I said could happen during dialysis and afterward? Well about three-quarters of them had happened that Monday night.

So, it was a bad morning. And, much to my dismay, one of my accountants was in to see me early and needed a decision.

Without going into the gory details, she needed to know how I wanted to account for an expense. I had a good feel for the issue and was able to make a decision pretty easily.

But, my mouth wasn't exactly working at full capacity yet.

What I intended to say: "Let's debit the prepaid accounts and put the offset in production."

What actually came out: "Let the prepaid offset put the official in production."

The accountant just sat there looking at me.

I said, "No, that's not right," and made a couple more attempts before finally getting it right.

I think I noticed her shaking her head slightly as she left my office.

Wherever possible, I would not make any major decisions if I wasn't feeling one hundred percent.

More important than making decisions, I tried to stay out of the limelight until I felt like a viable human being again. That sometimes meant avoiding contact with other people in the morning.

But, my dedication never faltered.

It was up to me to make sure I put in whatever effort was necessary to get the job done, regardless of how I felt. And that's what I did.

Fact is, most days, my strategy was to bury myself in my work and bring an intensity to my meetings, both as a way of getting my job done well and to keep from focusing on my dialysis-related ills.

I would use my not feeling well to my advantage, if you can believe that. Whenever I got a wave of nausea or an overriding urge to take a nap, I used the intensity of that feeling to refocus on whatever I was doing.

In other words, even on really bad days, focusing on my work acted as a cure for not feeling well. I was using work to *help* me live with dialysis.

The Cultural Void

Okay, you want to know what really ticks me off about this whole dialysis thing?

It's that, before I started dialysis, I was a *happening* dude.

Cool? Hah. My picture was in the dictionary under "cool."

I was super cool. I was street cool. I was…

Wait a minute. There's that laughing again.

All right, all right. Maybe I wasn't that cool. But I had a good sense of culture. I knew what was going on socially. Then those darn treatments came along.

They soak up too much of my time to maintain my cool factor.

More laughing?

Okay, well, maybe I wasn't cool at all.

In fact, you might say that culturally, I was a clueless knucklehead.

My idea of being up-to-speed was getting a newsletter from AARP.

But, I'm here to tell you that being on dialysis doesn't exactly help with staying current on culture. I mean, in addition to working full time and spending four to four-and-a-half hours three times per week dealing with your treatment means chances are pretty great you will be even more out-of-touch than you were before—a scary prospect.

The scientific{?}discussion about feeling old and grumpy is directly related to this cultural void.

In the last couple of years before retiring, while I was still on dialysis, I started to feel completely behind the times culturally.

After all, a big part of being successful in business is developing interpersonal relationships.

The ability to relate to people in a large corporation is often a critical part of getting the job done. It's not like understanding business issues; I never had a problem with that.

Being able to relate to people on a personal level often involves discussing subjects that fall under the wide umbrella of "culture." And remember, the great majority of the people who I usually came in contact with were significantly younger than I was. As a result, I had some difficulty staying current.

And, yes, I'm going to attribute part of the blame for my cultural ineptitude to being on dialysis. How do you like them apples?

I mean, how are you supposed to be "with-it" when these treatments take up so much of your time?

Being with-it was *never* my forte, but I do think my ability to stay current got worse after the start of the Big D.

In fact, there were times when I felt like about the least cool person on the planet.

One time, a friend of mine in the office told me that she bought tickets to an Opeth concert for her son's birthday.

She described Opeth as being a "Swedish death metal group."

It took me a while to realize that she wasn't kidding.

A Swedish death metal group, huh?

I feel old just saying that.

Around that same time, some people in the office (again, mostly younger) were talking about concerts they had attended recently. Fortunately, not everyone limited their taste to Swedish death metal music.

Still, I have to admit that I felt a little lost in the discussion.

I hadn't even heard of a single group they were mentioning.

They must have sensed my bewilderment, and I admitted that I hadn't been to a concert in a while.

They wanted details. "How long of 'a while' are we talking about here?" someone asked.

"Well, a while-while. You know, quite a while," I said evasively.

"What was the last concert you went to?"

I had to think hard, but I finally confessed it was Art Garfunkle in 1973.

When I said that, they all looked at me like I should have been sitting on a park bench somewhere with a blanket over my legs, sipping from a flask full of hot toddy.

Nobody said anything, but some of the people in the group looked like they didn't even know who Art Garfunkle was.

Another factor that fed into my lack of cultural awareness was my profession.

I was in corporate finance, not the hippest of roles you can play in a big company.

If you get a bunch of finance people together, it won't exactly result in a fun-loving, happy-go-lucky group.

Our idea of a good time is boning up on the latest depreciation tables.

I once actually had a lengthy argument with another executive about the use of net present value in preferred stock return calculations—earth-shattering subject matter.

We "finance types" did actually have social gatherings every once in a while.

One time, a bunch of finance associates went to an upscale Italian restaurant downtown for a holiday get-together. The place had two stories and we had rented out the top floor.

I arrived at the party and walked up to some of my fellow finance friends. One guy was telling what he thought was an outrageously funny story.

I got there mid-story, but he was saying something like:

"AND THIS GUY ASKED ME FOR TOTAL LIABILITIES WHEN HE REALLY ONLY NEEDED CURRENT LIABILITIES, HA HA HA HA HA HA..." as he was going into near hysterics.

I was like, take me now, Lord.

Later, it looked like a square eyeglass convention, with a bunch of finance people intently discussing current business issues.

I went over to the rail that overlooked the first floor dining room.

"Stop talking about business or I'm going to jump," I said.

They all stopped their conversation midstream and looked at me.

I was mentally going through what I thought the responses were in their minds.

I estimated that fifty percent thought I was right and were willing to stop talking business; forty percent were hoping I'd fulfill my promise and jump, thinking it would liven up the evening; and ten percent were pissed that I interrupted their conversation and wanted to push me over.

Anyway, as a group, they all sheepishly agreed that this was, after all, a party and that we should at least make an attempt to discuss some subject—any subject—other than business.

The party went pretty well for a while. Everyone loosened up, talking about their kids' sports teams or a movie they had seen recently—normal human being stuff. Very encouraging.

Later in the evening, however, I overheard a small group, made up of many of the same people as I had threatened earlier, discussing debits and credits in international accounting rules.

I just walked away shaking my head, thinking…hopeless. Being un-cool must be a *requirement* for working in finance.

So, I didn't get a lot of help from my peers in trying to solve my cultural knuckleheadedness.

The growing importance of *social media* in business added to my feeling of falling behind the times.

A big part of my job involved working with my company's marketing department.

Marketing people, in case you don't know, are usually among the youngest, hippest, most "with-it" folks around in a big company.

In marketing, associates have to stay up to date on all the latest trends as well as uses of different media types to reach their company's target customers.

As social media became more important as an advertising vehicle, I was suddenly surrounded by more and more savvy, smart, and, yes, cool individuals, which, of course, made me look even more ancient by comparison.

Now, I have to say that these marketing folks were more than patient with me in explaining the ins and outs of all this new media. (They sort of had to be, since I was in charge of their budget, but let's not dilute the compliment.)

The head of the digital media buying group took me through all of her recommendations very carefully. She was very patient when I needed extra clarification, but every once in a while she gave me a look that said, "What is this, bring your dinosaur to work week?"

Social and digital media are unique in that people you work with participate *personally* as well as in a business sense. Much to my distress, I found that most of my business associates were conversant in Facebook, Twitter, Groupon, and the like because they all had their own accounts.

For the longest time, I was completely left behind in conversations about these things.

It was *really* distressing when I found out that the wise guy friend of mine, who was actually a little older than me, was up to speed on social media as well.

I was with a group of people in a pre-meeting conversation that somehow drifted into the topic of digital media. People were talking about their Facebook activities, tossing around words and phrases that I knew nothing about.

My buddy waltzes in, and I thought, ah, at last someone else in my age group. He and I can commiserate on our lack of understanding about these things and talk about something to which the two of us can relate like maybe varicose veins or the cost of a postage stamp.

But nooo. He jumped right into the digital conversation.

"Yeah, the other day my wife was upset that I didn't 'Like' her post, so I went off and worked my Farmville, updated my profile, and searched out a few new apps," he said.

I just sat there staring at him.

He noticed my stunned expression and said, "What? Haven't you planted anything in Farmville lately?"

I just shook my head and pretended to understand what was being discussed until the meeting started and we could talk about work again.

Even talking about current TV shows would leave me in the dust.

Since I don't watch television during my treatments, again, I'm at a disadvantage when this subject comes up.

Once, I was having lunch with a group of associates in my organization, and they were talking up the latest reality shows, which, I guess you have to follow from the first episode to understand what's going on.

This was another situation that made me feel completely left out.

I thought, geez, am I the only one who doesn't know about these reality shows? I'm going to have to start watching something other than *The Simpsons* and reruns of *Sanford and Son*.

Sometimes, I would actually try to *hide* my lack of cultural awareness.

One time, some marketing folks came bounding into my office all excited. They were proposing a potential deal with Ryan Sheckler.

I tried to match their excitement and said, "Wow, really? Ryan Sheckler? Sounds like it has great potential. Let me see a draft of the contract when it's ready."

When they left, I ran out to my assistant.

"Who's Ryan Sheckler?" I asked.

(Of course a potential deal like that underwent a lot of scrutiny before getting approved.)

My assistant told me that Ryan Sheckler was a skateboarder, which explained why I had never heard of him. But apparently, he's very popular with the younger crowd.

Later that day, I was speaking to a large group of people, and in an effort to show that I was a with-it dude, I proudly mentioned that we were working on a potential deal with "Brian Selzer." Then, I smiled knowingly.

Instead of the positive uproar that I expected, I got a bunch of confused looks.

My assistant was in the crowd, and she slyly made her way to where I was standing and whispered, "It's *Ryan Sheckler*, you tool."

"Okay," I said, quickly trying to slough over my mistake, "next on the agenda…"

Retirement

Mid-year in 2011, my company offered early retirement to everyone over a certain age who had more than the minimum number of years of service.

At first, like an idiot, I started mentally going through the associates that I knew who were going to be eligible.

Then the light bulb went on.

Holy crap, I thought. *I'm* eligible.

Of course, your mind goes in a hundred directions in situations like that, but fortunately, I had a few months to decide whether or not I was going to retire.

I talked to many people who were astounded that I was even hesitating with the decision. The early retirement offer was very generous and included a full pension.

And, those who knew of my personal circumstances were even more amazed that I wasn't dancing in the halls.

"Are you kidding me?" one of them said. "No more dialysis and work. What's the problem?"

They had a point. I mean, by all rights, this should have been a complete no-brainer.

And yet, when the time came to make a decision, I still had a hard time pulling the trigger.

My life was so centered around my job that I worried about filling the void that would be left by not working.

And, I worried about being home more often and how that would affect my wife.

As a friend of mine, whose husband had recently retired put it:

"Having your husband retired is like having a piano in the kitchen. It's great having a piano, but no one wants it in the kitchen."

Anyway, to make a long and torturous story short, I did end up taking early retirement.

In terms of timing, my boss and I agreed that I would finish out the year, so at the time, I had about three months to continue working and pondering the unknown ahead of me.

The very day that I decided to retire, I found my stress level at work had significantly diminished. I obviously still wanted to do my job well, but suddenly business problems that used to send me up the wall and across the ceiling were just rolling off my shoulders.

As I was nearing the end of the year and getting closer to actually retiring, a few potential headlines were popping into my head for my forthcoming post-retirement days.

Maybe it would be:

SMOOTH, ISSUE-FREE RETIREMENT ENSUES

But, I thought there was also a possibility of:

DRIVEN CRAZY BY RETIREMENT: INSANE FORMER EXECUTIVE CLAIMS TO BE A TEAPOT

Or, perhaps:

WIFE OF RETIRED EXECUTIVE FOUND CHASING HIM OUT OF THE HOUSE WITH AN AXE

To put it mildly, there was a high degree of uncertainty about my future while I was still in my pre-retirement days.

One comforting factor for me was that there were many other associates in the same boat—people who had accepted the early retirement package and were nervous about retiring. So I had a lot of company and lots of folks with whom I could commiserate.

As you might expect, there were a wide variety of reactions among those preparing for the end of their working days.

Some were thrilled.

"Can you believe we get to retire early?" said one guy. "Best news I've had since the push-up bra was invented."

Some were anticipating their next job.

"Tell me how you think this sounds," another associate said. "Welcome to Wal-Mart. Need a shopping cart today?"

Others were just plain terrified.

"What am I going to do?" said yet another associate who was near retirement. "If I'm hanging around the house all day, my wife will want me to finish all the things I've been working on for the last ten years."

I could definitely relate and probably shared a little of each of their thoughts. My main line of thinking was running along three parts:

I was part excited about not having to deal with work while on dialysis any more.

I was partly anticipating potential new projects to work on.

And I was part terrified about being unable to fill my time and potentially driving my family crazy. And, as I mentioned, burying myself in my work was a way of not focusing on my dialysis-related miseries.

The last three months went by very fast and before I knew it, the time had come.

So, here I was. Officially retired. And I have to say, the first few months were pretty smooth.

I found the key to a good retirement is staying busy. In fact, for the first couple of months, there was very little down time when I was thinking, okay, what am I going to do now?

And, I avoided falling into the abyss of television.

Some retirees that I know started watching TV during the day—something that you can't do while working full time.

These recent retirees quickly started getting caught up in the cadence of daily shows and suddenly felt like they couldn't miss the next episode of their favorite program.

It's kind of like mental quicksand.

We established a hard rule in our house: the TV stays off until the afternoon news, at four to five in the evening

Regarding dialysis, I wanted to change my schedule after I retired to start getting my treatments first thing in the morning. My experience had been that early morning treatments were easier on my body. Having treatments in the evening after a stressful day in the office seemed to magnify the dialysis side effects.

When I had a day off while I was working, I would always try to change my treatment schedule to the early morning shift, so I had a good feel for what morning treatments were like.

I was a little concerned that there wouldn't be a slot for me on the "first shift" at my center, but when I asked about it, the charge nurse said, "Sure. No problem. We can't fill the chairs on the morning shift. Nobody wants it."

I was amazed, but, as it turns out, the first shift in the dialysis center looked like a convention of recent retirees.

The patients on the morning shift consisted of a handful of guys in my age group who were used to getting up early and who had years of experience with the grueling schedule of having dialysis after working all day.

We all had a lot in common, and we all agreed that we wanted to get our treatment done as early as possible and have the rest of the day to ourselves.

And we all arrive at the center well before our scheduled treatment time—sometimes even before the staff arrives.

Seems the punctuality of a career of working full time is now hard-wired into our brains.

On a typical dialysis day, you can find the bunch of us recent retiree patients sitting in our cars in the parking lot of the dialysis center listening to our radios, waiting for the sleepy staff to arrive.

"We should give you guys a key and let you come in and set up the machines," said one attendant.

So, now I get my treatment first thing in the morning, and afterward, I'm not nearly as physically spent as I was in the evening during my working days.

How are things as far as the home life goes after retiring?

Well, at the end of the first month, my wife was pondering what her life had been like over the past thirty days.

"My life hasn't really changed that much, except that you're always here," she said.

Hmmm. If I dig deep enough, I'm sure I can find something positive in there somewhere.

"Oh geez," she said. "That didn't come out right."

In general, retirement has gone much better than I expected. I have found that the key to making it work is staying busy and not letting my brain just rot away.

I have filled my time between working my investments, exercising, playing tennis, reading, writing, gardening, running chores, chasing the cat, and watching *The Doodlebops* with my grandson.

And I haven't even been chased by anyone wielding an axe.

At least, not yet…

Medical

It was my first hospital stay after starting dialysis. The doctor was in the room discussing dialysis basics.

Toward the end of the conversation he said, "The key to doing well on dialysis is being compliant. You know, doing what you're supposed to do, following the rules."

My wife just looked at me. It was a moment of stunned realization. She finally found her voice.

"Uh oh," she said.

Following rules, you see, is not exactly one of my strong points.

Or, as my wife claims: "When you think a rule is stupid, you figure it must not apply to you."

So true.

She sensed a real danger if we were going to be relying on me being compliant and sticking to the rules to stay healthy.

I also hate, Hate, HATE being told what to do—a trait which I think is strongly related to my dislike of rules.

Some people might describe my being this way as having a strong sense of individualism.

Others might call it a personality defect.

Whatever. As far back as I can remember, when someone ordered me to do something, or told me I *had* to do it, I immediately became just as likely to do the exact opposite.

In business, there would be absolute hell to pay if anyone told me we were doing something a certain way "because that's the way we've always done it."

I can't even type that now without practically breaking the keyboard.

Whenever someone tells me I can't do something, or even worse, says it's against the rules, my evil twin takes over and starts plotting ways to get around the way it "should" be done.

My tendency to ignore or intentionally violate rules started very young.

I was the kind of kid who would have put a peanut butter sandwich in the VCR just to see what would happen.

Except, of course, there were no VCRs when I was that age.

When my mother wanted me to learn how to play the guitar, I left to go to the lesson, hid the guitar in the front bushes, and went to play basketball with my friends at the schoolyard instead.

Growing up in New York, I had a group of what I affectionately call "hoodlum friends."

We never did anything real serious, like rob a bank, but we were a bunch of adolescents with no money, constantly on the lookout for an opportunity to do something cool. And no rules were going to stand in our way.

We would jump the turnstiles to get a free subway ride, go places we weren't supposed to go, whatever.

I even remember a local merchant chasing my friend and me up the street because we had tried to steal a *Playboy* magazine.

Some of our hoodlum group even figured a way to sneak into Shea Stadium and watch baseball games for free.

In the old setup at Shea, there was a utility building just behind the visitor's bullpen. It was just the right height that one of us could be lifted by the others to get on the roof.

Once one of us was on the roof, we would just pull the others up. Then we were able to climb into the seating and, voilà, we were in the park for free.

(I found it interesting that a few years later, I went back to the stadium, and the roof of the utility building had fencing and barbed wire on it. Guess our secret was out.)

Most of my hoodlum friends and I all got ourselves straightened out by the time opportunities for college came about, and many of us became upstanding citizens later in life. Go figure.

My dislike of authority started way back in school. It sometimes had a lasting impact on my relationship with teachers.

I remember one of my middle school teachers, Miss Bell. She was very authoritarian and wanted everybody to sit still and only speak when spoken to.

I was not exactly her favorite student. In fact, if she saw me in the street, she would have had a hard time resisting the urge to run me down with her car.

Man had just walked on the moon for the first time (no snickering about age allowed) and in celebration of the event, Miss Bell wanted us to use words related to space travel in a sentence. I guess she was trying to improve our verbal acuity.

The next word was "launch" and she called on me.

I thought for a minute, then I said, "When I saw the questions on your quiz last week, it made me want to launch."

There was some laughter in the background, but Miss Bell just gave me an icy stare.

"I'm not sure I understand your use of the word," she said.

Ever helpful, and never one to leave well enough alone, I went on to explain.

"You know, upchuck, hurl, blow chunks…that kind of launch."

Now, there was a lot of laughter, but Miss Bell was staring at me with a look of pure fury. She was so mad, she quit on the word usage exercise right then and there.

Later in the school year, whenever she started to forget why she hated me so much, one of my friends would remedy the situation by running toward the classroom door in the middle of class with his hands over his mouth, saying, "Ooooh, Miss Bell, I think I'm gonna launch…"

Then, they would run out into the hall toward the boys' room.

Needless to say, my relationship with Miss Bell was never very good that year.

My transgressions got a little more serious as I got older. When I was in my mid-teens, I didn't think I should have to wait to drive until I was old enough to get a license. So, I took my father's car without his knowing about it, went out for a little joy ride, and got into a fender-bender accident.

There were a little more serious consequences for that one.

My tendency to disregard rules and protocol continued into adulthood.

Again, nothing you need to call 9-1-1 over.

I just really get roiled if I disagree with the principle involved in a rule or even just a basic way of doing something.

As part of my job, I was always looking to change processes that had been done the same way for a long time.

As I mentioned earlier, when I first started dialysis, I didn't exactly see eye-to-eye with the doctor about when I could go back to work after my first hospital stay.

The doctor pointed out that, right before I started dialysis, I was a pretty sick guy. I didn't really know what was wrong with me and, like most guys, I waited way too long to seek medical help.

When the doctor and nurse saw the results of my initial blood test, they almost fainted. My creatine and blood urea nitrogen (BUN), both of which reflect on kidney function, were *way* out of whack.

So, after my hospital stay was over, the good doctor wanted me to take some time to recover before going back to work. The real problem came when he suggested a four- to six-week recovery time.

I asked, "How did you decide on that amount of time?"

He said, "That's the usual amount of time that we recommend."

Uh-oh. Wrong answer.

"Sure Doc, no problem. Makes perfect sense to me," said Evil Bob.

So, I took my *one* week off, and back to work I went.

Here's the kicker to my living a lifetime of non-compliance:

I'm a *compliant* dialysis patient.

It comes as something of a surprise to me, but I actually do what I'm supposed to on the dialysis regimen.

The people in my center actually use me as an example of how to live well on dialysis. Being used as an example of the right way to behave is definitely something new for me.

The patient whose girlfriend ratted him out to the doctor? The staff was sitting him near me purposely, hoping some of my good behavior would rub off on him.

So, what caused the turnaround in my attitude toward rules and compliance, you might ask?

Well, through trial and error, I came to realize that I'm really only hurting myself if I don't follow the diet guidelines, watch the fluid intake, be careful of excess sodium, etc.

The consequences for a dialysis patient not behaving diet-wise range from torturous treatments (and the treatments are not really pleasant to begin with) to serious health problems in addition to kidney failure.

So, the basis of my getting along okay medically after several years of being on dialysis runs somewhat counter to my natural personality.

I finally found a set of rules I can follow.

Doctors

Do you know how to keep a doctor from drowning?

You take your foot off his head.

Whoa, there's a little more venom in that than I intended, but it brings across the general idea that doctors are not exactly my favorite people.

Now, if the doctors who treat me at the dialysis center are reading this—love y'all, mean it.

Seriously, saying that I don't like doctors is a gross generalization. It would be more accurate to say that I don't like *some* doctors.

Or, the percentage of people who are doctors who I don't like is higher than that of the general population.

Wow, I sounded like a doctor just then.

My gripes with doctors fall into two general categories.

Gripe # 1: As smart as they might be, doctors can't communicate worth spit.

They may have studied hard in college and aced all their medical courses, but most doctors act like they skipped "Conversation 101."

Sometimes communication problems result from a combination of doctors having such a powerful influence in our lives, and their being, as a group, some of the most clueless creatures who have ever walked upright on this earth.

What really sends me into orbit is when a doctor looks to *me* for answers that I think he/she should be providing.

I was working with a nephrologist when I was in the latter stages of kidney failure.

For the purposes of anonymity, we'll refer to this kidney doctor as "Dr. Smith."

As in *Lost in Space*. Very appropriate.

Since this was my first experience with End Stage Renal Disease (ESRD), I was far from an expert in understanding what my body was going through.

I had been to Dr. Smith's office for some blood tests, and he called me the next day.

"It's Dr. Smith."

"Yes doctor."

"Your potassium's high."

At the time, I didn't know potassium from bubble gum, so I waited for him to continue.

Nothing.

Finally, I said, "Can you tell me a little bit more?"

He said, "Yes, your reading came in too high."

"I gathered that, but what does that mean?"

"It means that your potassium level is too high."

At this point, I was starting to twitch.

Then he said, "Why do you think your potassium is too high?"

Evil Bob's smartass attitude started to rear its ugly head.

"I don't know. Why do *you* think it's too high?" I said.

"I don't know," he said.

"Oh, okay, well, it's been really nice talking to you, Doc. Don't be a stranger." And I hung up.

This was probably when I first started thinking that you had to fail an intelligence test to become a doctor.

Dr. Smith called me back later and wanted me to retake the test. But did he really have to torture me first?

Another time I went to a dermatologist who looked at a spot on my skin.

"What's this?" he said.

I said, "Don't *you* know what it is?"

"Looks like an Actinic Kerotosis."

I said, "Ah, that was my next guess. Right after *Little Red Spot*."

Another time, a primary care physician took my blood pressure, and it was a little high.

He said, "Hmm, your blood pressure's a little high. Any idea why?"

Then, we had a little back-and-forth about who should really know why it was high.

Finally, he said, "Let me take it again."

Lo and behold, it was even higher.

I said, "At least this time I *know* why it's high."

After a few of these physician encounters, I was about at the point that if another doctor looked to *me* for a diagnosis, I was going to jump off the nearest ledge.

When you think about it, it's pretty rare to be around someone who can cure you *and* make you sick all at the same time.

Gripe # 2: As a group, doctors have an insufferable superiority complex.

Despite their inability to communicate, somewhere along the line many doctors come to see themselves as superior to those of us who are not in the medical profession.

Now, I understand that doctors go through rigorous education and training programs. But do they really think they're the only ones who are smart?

This feeling of superiority on the part of doctors frequently manifests itself by keeping patients waiting for interminably long periods of time when they have an appointment in their office.

I know, I know, sometimes the doctor's prior appointments take longer than they expected. Obviously, there's nothing you can do about that.

But, I can't tell you how many times I've seen doctors goofing around in their offices or making time with a nurse while a patient (particularly this patient) was waiting.

You just get the feeling that they think their time is more valuable than ours.

Sometimes, a doctor's incredibly high opinion of himself comes across in a routine conversation.

One time I was having a procedure done in a hospital, and I was on my gurney waiting to go under in the prep room.

I had a great nurse who was waiting by my side.

This doctor comes in from the other room and stops to chat with my nurse.

I didn't catch the whole conversation, but I tuned in about when he was saying, "...And I brought my car in for service, and this guy in overalls comes over and says, 'What can I do for you, buddy?'"

Then he paused for impact, looking at the nurse.

"Can you believe that?" he continued. "*Buddy*. Can you believe he called me buddy? ME? I said to him, 'Don't call me buddy.'"

The nurse just stared at him.

At this point, of course, I had to pipe in.

"I don't know, I've been called a lot worse," I said.

The doctor gave a start, as if he was not even aware that I was there.

"Anybody ever call you jerk-weed?" I asked him.

He looked taken aback.

"Um...well...no, certainly not."

"No? How about numb-nuts?"

The nurse had her hand over her mouth and was suppressing a laugh.

"Of course not."

"Needle-nose? Knucklehead? Butt-munch?"

At this point, he gave me one final dirty look and made to leave.

"I'll catch up with you later," he said to the nurse.

She was still trying not to laugh in the doctor's face so she just nodded. But, of course, I had to say goodbye.

"Later dude…er pal…er homey…I mean… goodbye, Doctor," I said formally.

He went off in a huff.

The nurse was laughing.

"Can you believe that pompous ass?" she said.

In fairness, because the subject matter about which we consult doctors is so serious—our health and our lives—a negative interaction with a doctor becomes magnified.

You might go into a meeting with your doctor feeling fairly neutral about physicians as a group only to come out feeling like you want their next convention to take place at the bottom of the ocean.

I've had a pretty good relationship with the doctors who have treated me *regularly* over the years. It seems to me that the doctors who only see you once or twice might tend to treat you like a number instead of a person.

I understand that medical schools are focused on providing technical training and education, but I think they should put more emphasis on the ability for their students to relate to people.

Maybe they could give the real bad cases personality transplants before unleashing them on the public.

Nurses/Attendants

Caretakers, Friends, Angels, Goddesses.

These are the words that describe the nurses and attendants who I've encountered during my life on dialysis.

As spotty as my relationship with doctors has been, I've developed a real bond with these caregivers.

You would think that doctors would be the front line in providing care with such a serious illness, but really it's the nurses and attendants at the dialysis centers who do much of the critical work.

During one treatment in a previous dialysis center, I had one of those infiltration episodes that I described earlier. One of the needles went right through the vessel, and before I knew it, my forearm looked like a bulldog had burrowed up under my skin.

I remember there was a young doctor subbing for the usual physician who did the rounds in that center. The guy looked like he was barely out of high school.

When I alerted the staff that the needle had infiltrated, the young doc came sauntering over for a look at my swollen arm.

"Wow," he said.

Eight years of medical school.

I could've gotten that from the guy who cuts my hair.

Anyway, the nurse in the center came over, brushed the kid-doctor aside, and went to work on my arm.

She applied ice to the swelling, slowly removed the infiltrated needle, and positioned my arm to set for a while. She returned shortly, carefully reinserted the needle at another site above the infiltration site, and a few minutes later, I was back in business, my treatment continuing.

During this entire process, the young doc was watching in amazement, as if he'd never seen a medical procedure before.

"Can I ask you a personal question?" I said, startling the guy a little.

"Uh… sure," he replied.

"How old are you?"

He looked a little uncertain that he wanted to answer, but finally he said, "Thirty-three."

I just nodded, muttered something under my breath about having underwear older than that, and went on with my treatment.

Dialysis patients spend a lot of time around these nurses and attendants, and sometimes they become like family. You get to know the nurses and attendants as well as co-workers you see every day for eight hours or more.

In addition to being the front line of your dialysis care, these are the folks who will be sticking you with two fifteen-gauge needles every other day.

Someone with that responsibility had better be someone you can trust.

The nurses and attendants are always present when you are sitting still for these wonderful treatments for three to four hours a pop. Sometimes, some restlessness can ensue. (On the part of the patient, that is.)

I remember one treatment where my blood pressure was doing a roller coaster ride. Too high one minute, too low the next.

My attendant was watching my BP carefully, but the combination of my going a little stir-crazy sitting in that chair for so long and the fact that I'm easily amused made me want to make a game of it.

She came over to check the BP again.

"Bob's pressure has been all over the board today, so let's see how it comes in now," I said in a low golf-broadcast voice, doing a play-by-play.

The attendant just looked at me with a little smirk.

The reading came in a little low, and the alarm went off.

"And, how about that?" I said to no one. "The kid manages the rare double, setting the alarm off for a high reading then a low reading on consecutive tries!"

And I did a version of a little break dance in my chair.

The attendant just shook her head but finally gave out a little laugh.

"Bob, I think dialysis is affecting your brain," she said.

"Hey, that's not true…well, okay maybe a little."

If and when there is a crisis during your treatment (seems like you never go very long without one), it's the nurses/attendants who react, giving you saline, stopping the bleeding, angling your head down, icing down the swelling, recommending hospitalization/psychiatric evaluation, whatever.

And, because you spend so much time with these individuals, your conversations can hit on a wide range of topics.

One time during a treatment, I had a lengthy exchange with the charge nurse and two attendants about our favorite weapons in *Angry Birds*.

"I like the yellow speed-birds," said one female attendant. "I just love hitting the screen and watching the birds cut those dirty pigs in half, ha ha ha."

One of the other patients, who didn't have the first clue what we were talking about, just looked at her with a little fear in his eyes.

"No, I like the big red cardinal birds," said the male attendant. "After all, it's not just about killing the pigs; it's causing destruction that gets you the big points. Besides, I always had a bit of a destructive streak anyway."

This caused me, the clueless patient, the other attendant, and the nurse to all look at the male attendant with a little fear.

The nurse voted for the multi-directional pelicans, claiming that your ability to maneuver those showed true skill in the game.

"Anybody can smash through things with those other birds," she said, looking at her co-workers doubtfully.

I just made a psshhh sound derisively.

"You guys don't know *Angry Birds* from *Smelly Turds*," I said. "The black bomb-bird rules. You can knock things down and blow them up all at the same time."

At this point, the other patient was looking like he'd just been beamed into the middle of an asylum.

"It pisses me off when all you get are those small cardinals," I continued. "They can't destroy crap."

We were continuing our pretty vocal discussion on this weighty issue when, unbeknownst to us, a district manager from the company that runs the dialysis center came in.

Before we even realized he was there, he had come up from behind and had overheard our conversation.

He gave a little <ahem> to announce his presence, making us all jump in unison. He was pretty formal looking in a suit and tie, carrying a clipboard.

We all turned around and looked at him, the center employees no doubt wondering if their goose was cooked and me wondering if he was going to have me transferred to a psych ward somewhere.

"I always preferred the egg-dropping bomb-birds, myself," he said. "You know if you position them correctly, they can destroy by jettisoning them strategically when they drop their egg?"

We all broke out laughing. Everyone except the other patient, who now looked like there was truly no hope.

Whenever a nurse or attendant from the dialysis center leaves, whether for another job, retirement, or whatever, we always bring them a little gift and exchange contact information.

We have stayed in contact with several of them years after they moved on.

Social Workers/Dieticians

Like the nurses/attendants, the social workers and dieticians (SW&D) are, for the most part, well-intentioned people looking out for your best interests.

Like with doctors, however, my relationship with the SW&Ds has been a little strained at times.

An unfortunate circumstance for the SW&Ds is that they have to do their jobs *while* their patients are undergoing dialysis treatments—not the most ideal time to have an in-depth conversation.

In addition, each of these employees carries a bit of professional baggage by the very nature of their job. And, I'll admit that my personality probably makes their duties even more difficult to perform.

Social workers need to talk to you about a lot of very personal information. Talking about myself personally was never something I was very good at, but I'm *really* bad when I am counting down the minutes for my dialysis treatment to be over.

Dieticians are in the unenviable position of being the enforcer of your renal dietary restrictions.

Both the social workers and the dieticians occasionally have to "lecture" their patients. Now, I never liked being lectured to start with. But lecturing me while I'm on dialysis? Not a very pleasant prospect.

Very similar to my relationship with doctors, I'm pretty good with the SW&D that I work with on a regular basis. You tend to get to know each other a little and that helps build a better rapport.

It's the substitutes, or, even worse, the SW&D who see you when you're visiting another center that I usually have problems with. These people tend to treat you like a number, which makes me a little nutty.

> I was traveling on vacation for a week and had three treatments scheduled at a dialysis center close to where I was staying. On my first of three sessions, this social worker came over and started asking me all kinds of questions that I didn't feel like answering.

> I got the feeling she was trying to change my life in one easy lesson. She started lecturing me about working too much, lifestyle, personal habits, yada, yada, yada.

> Finally, I had had enough, and I pretended to fall asleep mid-sentence.

> I said, "Well, I like to keep up the pace by sustaining my lifestyle and making sure................................."

> I closed my eyes and let my head fall back.

I could sense that she was a little stumped on what to do.

After a lengthy pause, she said softly, "Bob?. Bob, are you okay?"

I just continued with my fake nap.

Eventually, she got up and left.

I kept my eyes closed for a while, but I peeked a little bit and the next time she was walking by, I suddenly opened my eyes, sat up, and continued my prior conversation right where I had left off.

"…that I continue to make progress both personally and professionally."

She stopped and looked at me. Again, not totally certain what to do, she made to come over to me three or four times, then decided against it and went to hide in the office.

On my second treatment, she got up the courage to try again, and I pulled my fake falling asleep mid-sentence act one more time.

I wasn't completely sure that she was buying the whole thing, but when I came back for my third and final treatment of the vacation week, she approached me with a lot of hesitation.

I, of course, acted like nothing was amiss.

"Oh, Hi! Good to see you. This week has really gone by fast, hasn't it?" I said, pleasant as all get out.

Then, after some small chitchat, she said, "Ummm... Bob, by any chance, have you ever been diagnosed with narcolepsy? You know, suddenly falling asleep, like in the middle of the day?"

I just laughed a little bit at first. Then I tried to explain the truth to the poor woman, but I started laughing even harder, and I couldn't stop. So, I never really got a clear explanation out to her, and eventually she went back to her office again, shaking her head.

I've been able to maintain a better relationship with dieticians over the years mainly because I'm generally compliant with my renal diet restrictions.

A couple of years ago, I did have an issue getting my phosphorous within an acceptable range. Since I am good about avoiding foods with high phosphorous content, my dietician thought the elevated reading might be related to the *Hectorol* dosage they were administering during my treatment.

Without getting too technical, dialysis patients are sometimes deficient in Vitamin D because we patients have to avoid dairy products, which are typically high in phosphorous. The problem with not consuming dairy is that the category is a good source of Vitamin D.

Vitamin D helps the body absorb calcium from the intestines into the blood. If the blood calcium level drops, the parathyroid gland can secrete excess hormones into the system to try to keep calcium and phosphorous in balance.

The side effect of low Vitamin D is that the blood can pull extra calcium out of the bones. This will cause both the phosphorous reading and PTH, measuring the amount of parathyroid hormone in your bloodstream, to be elevated in routine blood tests.

Some patients are given Hectorol as a substitute for Vitamin D, but until the dosage and frequency are adjusted correctly, the result can be some elevated phosphorous readings.

Anyway, my regular dietician and I were pretty much on the same page that my elevated phosphorous readings were caused by an incorrect Hectorol dosage and that we needed to work on an adjustment.

Unfortunately, my regular dietician went out on maternity leave, and her substitute was a know-it-all type who didn't know about the Hectorol issue. This temporary dietician immediately started lecturing me about the evils of not watching the phosphorous in my diet.

The situation presented me with a "perfect storm" of things that stick in my craw.

By nature, I don't like know-it-all types.

I hate being lectured.

And, perhaps worst of all, I don't like when someone implies that I'm not compliant with my diet, when I put so much effort into toeing the line.

So, after Ms. Know-It-All Dietician came to a break in her lecture on my phosphorous, she looked at me defiantly and said, "So, what do you have to say for yourself?"

I just looked at her silently for a minute, then I blurted out, "Corny Dogs!"

She blinked her eyes a few thousand times.

"What?" she said.

"Corny Dogs!" I repeated.

After a moment she said, "What about corny dogs??"

"Corny dogs are the culprit," I said forcefully.

She scrunched up her face and said, "What are you talking about?"

"It was the State Fair," I said, adding a flare of drama. "I shouldn't have gone, but I did. I knew that if I went, I wouldn't be able to resist the corny dogs. They have tons of sodium and are loaded with phosphorous, but when I got there, I knew that I'd be their slave."

She was just looking at me.

"The moment I got there," I went on rapid-fire, "it was clear that I really only wanted those corny dogs, and I was driving everyone else nuts. Finally, the people I was with just relented, and I ran up to the corny dog stand, looking like I hadn't eaten in a month, and ordered up two big ones, and the guy behind the stand just looked at me, and finally I said, 'Where's my dogs, man?' and he said, 'Sir, don't you think nine o'clock in the morning is a little early for corny dogs?' I said, 'I need the dogs, man!' So he had to cook some because they hadn't started cooking them yet, I mean, he was just finishing breakfast, but finally he brought them to me. I said 'Oh thanks, brother' and he just muttered something in response, although I'm pretty sure I heard the word 'schmuck' in there somewhere, and I wolfed down those dogs, and, oh I forgot, just in case they didn't have quite enough sodium, I practically drowned them in mustard, and then of course, later on, I had to go for a jog because these things have like one hundred percent fat content. But boy, I felt fulfilled after having those dogs. You ever feel totally fulfilled? Never mind, but I'm sure that was why my reading was high, that's got to be it..."

She was standing there in stunned silence.

Then, I'm sure she figured she no longer cared about this nut-job's phosphorous and quickly moved on to another patient.

Fortunately, my regular dietician returned and we picked up right where we left off with a pretty good relationship.

I know social workers and dieticians are all trying to help their patients. And I know that I'm not always the easiest person for them to work with. But all I can say is that I'm doing my best to get along.

And, for any SW&Ds in other centers that I might be visiting in the future, I apologize in advance for my behavior. But, look at the bright side.

I'll only be in *your* center temporarily...

Crazy Behavior

The reason I'm including this in the Medical section is that I'm convinced dialysis is responsible my sometimes crazy behavior.

That's right. I'm blaming it all on these treatments.

So, I'm sure you're wondering, does that mean my behavior was completely normal before I started dialysis?

Hey, work with me here. I've got a convenient excuse and I'm running with it.

The way I figure it, the causes of this "off-kilter" behavior are two-fold: physical and physiological.

How's that for trying to make a cockamamie theory sound legitimate by tossing around some big words?

The physical part is related to being confined to those treatment chairs for very long periods of time. It's only normal to want to let loose after sitting in one spot for four hours, right?

> In one of the rare instances after a treatment when I felt well enough to accompany my wife to the grocery store, she was really wondering whether these dialysis sessions were making me soft-in-the-head.

> Okay, okay, maybe it's soft<u>er</u>.

She made the brave decision to take me along, and we were going to one of these high-class stores; you know, the ones that fancy up their décor a bit so they can charge higher prices?

I had just finished a treatment and was feeling pretty good, relatively speaking, that is.

As part of the ambience of the store, there was top-notch music playing in the background, as opposed to the stale old "elevator music" you normally hear in some of the older stores.

To my wife's misfortune, the song that was playing when we first walked in was a real rocking dance song, the kind that makes you want to boogie right on the spot.

And, remember, I had just been sitting still in a chair for more than four hours. It's hard to describe the restlessness that I was feeling.

So, I grabbed my wife and started to dance right in front of everybody in the front of the store.

Before she really knew what was going on, I went through a series of dance steps and used my momentum to twirl her under my arm.

Then, she got her wits about her and tried to stop me, but I really had the rhythm going and kept right on dancing.

Finally, she had had enough, threw my arms away, stomped her feet, and yelled, "STOP THAT, YOU LUNATIC!"

Everyone was staring, so, to make matters worse, I calmly walked over to her and said softly, "How many times have I asked you not to make a scene in public?"

When I looked into her eyes just then, I saw me dead.

Occasionally, the urge to misbehave can hit you mid-treatment. I mean, you try to keep yourself busy as much as possible to make the time go by, but with three treatments per week, you're bound to have some periods when you're bored and there's nothing going on.

One time, I was on a weekend vacation, visiting an out-of-town center for one treatment—fertile territory for bad behavior.

To make the situation worse, the dietician in this center, who I obviously didn't know from a hole in the wall, started lecturing me about one of my blood test readings that had been sent over from my usual center.

I really wasn't paying attention, and in response to one of her questions, I spouted off a phrase in French.

I hadn't taken French since high school so, strictly translated, my words were complete nonsense, something like, "I want to rebuild your grandmother's shoes."

The dietician looked at me like I was totally cracked.

Imagine that.

She tried repeating her question, and I kept answering with the same tricked-out, broken French answer.

Finally she gave up, figuring the conversation was going nowhere, and walked away shaking her head.

On the physiological causes of crazy behavior, I got a hint that something was going to be amiss early on in my dialysis life.

Shortly after starting dialysis, I went back to the hospital for a follow-up meeting with my doctor. In the course of the session, he said he also wanted me to see the hospital dietician.

The doctor left when the dietician arrived. She started to ask me a bunch of relatively routine questions.

After some preliminary inquiries, she asked, "Do you ever get the urge to eat dog food?"

I just sat there looking at her, expecting there to be a punch line.

Then I realized that she was serious, and I said, "Well…uh… no…although my cat's chewy treats make a killer crouton, ha ha ha."

She just looked exasperated.

"How about dirt?" she continued.

"Dirt?"

"Yes, dirt."

"Are you asking if I ever want to eat dirt?"

"Yes."

I couldn't even come up with a smartass remark about that one.

"Uh, no, not lately," I said.

"Laundry detergent? Clay? Cement?"

Again, I just stared at her, dumbfounded.

Then I said, "Well, I have to admit, my wife's fabric softener does look pretty tasty." Then I laughed to show that I was kidding.

Not even a smirk from the dietician, however.

"I'm asking you these questions very seriously," she said.

"Okay, then no. No, I never get the urge to eat laundry detergent, clay, cement, Mr. Clean, or Murphy's Oil Soap. No. I guess if I want a snack, though, I can always just run out to the local hardware store, ha ha ha."

She looked down and took a deep breath.

"The reason I'm asking is that dialysis can bring on a condition known as *pica*. Sometimes, the renal diet can result in a mineral deficiency, which can cause the onset of this illness. Pica can result in the desire to consume non-food items," she said.

"Well that would have been helpful information to start with. I was beginning to think I was being punked with a hidden camera or something."

I admitted that it seemed dialysis *was* doing some funky things to my senses.

Food didn't smell the same or taste the same.

Fortunately, I hadn't had any symptoms of pica, but when this dietician was telling me about it, I started worrying about what would happen if I developed the disease.

I had visions of attending a formal dinner party at someone's house, with everyone dressed to the nines, and me excusing myself from the table to have a shot at the dog's bowl in the kitchen.

Or, I imagined being at an outdoor cookout with everyone gathered around the barbeque and me over eyeing the dirt in the garden.

The potential scenarios were endless.

So, if you're on dialysis and you notice that your behavior is becoming a little whacked, relax, there may be a medical reason for it.

And, if you know someone on dialysis, don't be too concerned if they act a little crazy at times.

But, you may want to keep the dog food in a safe place...

Peeing

So, this nun comes charging into the head priest's office in a Catholic school, right?

She says, "Father, I was walking down the hall, and I heard a commotion in the boys' room."

The priest says, "Yes, what happened?"

She says, "Well, I looked in to see what was going on, and three boys were in there competing to see who could pee farthest up on the wall."

The priest says, "Interesting, what did you do?"

She says, "I hit the ceiling."

Ah, jokes about peeing. I know there is a stream of good ones out there.

Hey, did I just say a "stream" of jokes about peeing? Now *that's* funny.

But, in all seriousness, here's the thing about peeing for dialysis patients: we don't.

That's right.

We don't pee.

Well, *most* dialysis patients who have been on the treatment for any length of time don't pee.

You see, urine is made by the kidneys, and when the kidneys don't work, the well eventually runs dry, so to speak—hence the need for dialysis patients to limit fluid intake.

The body eliminates excess fluid largely through urination.

Excess fluid may not sound like a big deal, but if fluid builds up in your heart or lungs, it will be a major problem.

Dialysis treatments remove excess fluid, but it is a really good idea to keep the intake down between sessions.

Because…well, because there's no peeing to relieve the overload.

Let me tell you, peeing is one of those things you take for granted until you don't do it anymore. I used to think, geez, what a pain it is to have to go all the time.

Now I think, ahhh, those were the good ole days.

Most people are really surprised when they learn that dialysis patients don't urinate. And, no, it's not like I stop strangers on the street and say, "Hey, guess what?"

But, you can tell someone about all the potential health pitfalls of kidney disease—you know, heart failure, anemia, calcification of your organs, etc. etc.—and their usual response will be a little "Aww" with a slight shrug of the shoulders.

But, tell them that you don't pee, and it's "What? You don't pee!? What do you mean you don't pee!?"—proving that everything is relative, and perspectives are all different.

I occasionally find myself thinking about peeing while I'm having my treatment.

(Hey, I told you, we have a lot of time to kill.)

The other day, I was thinking about some of the famous *places* that I've peed.

The list was quite distinguished.

It included multiple state houses, stadiums, museums, and arenas.

For some extra fun, I started thinking about all the times I've peed outdoors or, even better, in public.

You may be aghast, but there are very few guys who haven't done it at one time or another. Modesty is not generally one of our notable qualities.

Some good news coming out of all this is that dialysis patients are great companions on long trips. We never have to look for a rest stop.

And if we go to the movies, we never have to worry about missing part of the film because of the extra-large Coke that we drank earlier.

How's that for looking at the bright side of things?

Conclusion

This book is largely based on being able to laugh at yourself and not taking life too seriously, even when the situation is dire.

When I told a fellow patient that I was writing a humorous book about dialysis, he said, "There is nothing funny about being on dialysis."

But, when I think about some of the situations that we patients are put in, there is fertile territory for comic relief. Besides, laughing is better than crying all the time. Crying can get embarrassing.

Nothing in this book should make you think that I do not take kidney failure seriously. Believe me, I do. I have to.

But if you are on dialysis, or know and love someone on dialysis, and any of the situations I describe in the book seem familiar, perhaps you might smile the next time they happen. If so, the effort of writing this book has been worthwhile.

The old cliché "Laughter is the best medicine" is one that I not only believe in, but one that I live by.

I truly hope that you've enjoyed this book and that perhaps I've brought a little sunshine into your day.

To my fellow dialysis patients: Our lives are hard…laugh harder.

Acknowledgements

I would be remiss if I didn't talk about the people in my life who have made being on dialysis livable, and who, by their patience and caring, made it possible for me to take a humorous look at this very serious situation.

I didn't talk about it much in the book, but after I first went on dialysis, my mother donated a kidney to me. The kidney lasted almost seventeen years, and they were some of the best years of my life. I honestly don't know if I could have advanced in my career the way I did if I was on dialysis at the time. The difficulty of doing so became clear when the kidney gave out and I had to combine work and my treatments.

Mom, words can't describe how appreciative I am about what you did for me. There's really no way that I can think of to thank you properly. You are truly a gift from God.

I speak of my wife Donna frequently in these pages. What I don't bring across is how important her ongoing support and love has been to managing this very difficult lifestyle. Baby, thank you for everything. My love for you knows no boundaries.

(Donna also had a significant role in editing the book.)

I also must say a few words about my family and friends. Everyone who knows about my situation, including my brother and two sisters, their spouses, my two children, their spouses, my cousins, and many of my friends all volunteered to be tested to see if they were potential kidney donors for me. There is no question in my mind that any one of them would have gladly been tested and donated if I had not stubbornly prevented it. It is a blessing to have you all in my life.

I also mention my assistant who worked for me before I retired. As you may have surmised, she was much more than just my assistant at work. She was also a major source of support and became one of my closest friends. And, yes, she also wanted to be tested.

It is with all this in mind that I can say that, despite being a victim of kidney failure, I consider myself to be one *extremely* lucky guy.

About the Author

Bob Northam recently retired from his position as vice president of finance for a Fortune 500 company. He has been a dialysis patient for a number of years. He and his wife Donna live in Texas. They have two adult children and one grandchild.

Made in the USA
Charleston, SC
02 November 2012